D0754114

INTERNAL FAMILY SYSTEMS THERAPY

THE GUILFORD FAMILY THERAPY SERIES
Michael P. Nichols, *Series Editor*
Alan S. Gurman, *Founding Editor*

Recent Volumes

INTERNAL FAMILY SYSTEMS THERAPY
Richard C. Schwartz

NORMAL FAMILY PROCESSES, Second Edition
Froma Walsh, EDITOR

CHANGING THE RULES: A CLIENT-DIRECTED APPROACH TO THERAPY
Barry L. Duncan, Andrew D. Solovey, and Gregory S. Rusk

TRANSGENERATIONAL FAMILY THERAPIES
Laura Giat Roberto

THE INTIMACY PARADOX: PERSONAL AUTHORITY IN THE FAMILY SYSTEM
Donald S. Williamson

HUSBANDS, WIVES, AND LOVERS:
THE EMOTIONAL SYSTEM OF THE EXTRAMARITAL AFFAIR
David J. Moultrup

MEN IN THERAPY: THE CHALLENGE OF CHANGE
Richard L. Meth and Robert S. Pasick,
with Barry Gordon, Jo Ann Allen, Larry B. Feldman, and Sylvia Gordon

FAMILY SYSTEMS IN MEDICINE
Christian N. Ramsey, Jr., EDITOR

NEGOTIATING PARENT–ADOLESCENT CONFLICT:
A BEHAVIORAL–FAMILY SYSTEMS APPROACH
Arthur L. Robin and Sharon L. Foster

FAMILY TRANSITIONS: CONTINUITY AND CHANGE OVER THE LIFE CYCLE
Celia Jaes Falicov, EDITOR

FAMILIES AND LARGER SYSTEMS:
A FAMILY THERAPIST'S GUIDETHROUGH THE LABYRINTH
Evan Imber-Black

Internal Family Systems Therapy

Richard C. Schwartz

The Guilford Press
New York   London

© 1995 The Guilford Press
A Division of Guilford Publications
72 Spring Street, New York, NY 10012
www.guilford.com

Printed in the United States of America

This book is printed on acid-free paper.

Last digit is print number: 18 17 16 15 14 13 12 11

Library of Congress Cataloging-in-Publication Data
Schwartz, Richard C.
     Internal family systems therapy / Richard C. Schwartz.
         p. cm. — (The Guilford family therapy series)
     Includes bibliographical references and index.
     ISBN 978-0-89862-273-7—ISBN 978-1-57230-272-3 (pbk.)
     1. Psychotherapy patients—Family relationships. 2. Multiple
personality. 3. Psychosynthesis. 4. Family—Psychological aspects.
5. Family psychotherapy. I. Title. II. Series.
RC489.F33S24 1995
616.89′14—dc20   94-21393
                                                        CIP

Acknowledgments

To adequately acknowledge my debt to the people whose help and ideas have influenced the internal family systems (IFS) model would take a book in itself. I am blessed to have encountered many guides along the way, and continue to rely on several of them.

My clients deserve most of the credit for this model, and yet I cannot thank them publicly by name. Often my role has been simply that of a journalist, recording the extrordinary things they discovered and reported to me. I can never fully appreciate the courage it took for many of them to enter and remain in what sometimes seemed an inner chamber of horrors or abyss of despair. They also taught me about my own inner world and how to live in it differently. I recommend that all therapists allow their clients to mentor them in the practice of psychotherapy and the living of life; it is an enlightening and transforming experience.

The colleagues, students, and workshop participants who have influenced the model, sometimes by simply mentioning a book or a method or by challenging an idea or technique that I had reified, are numerous. Some among them have devoted much of their professional energy to the model's development and have made special contributions. Deborah Gorman-Smith has been a partner in exploration over the past several years. Her sensitivity to issues facing survivors of sex abuse and to the therapist–client relationship have enriched the model enormously, and her relentless skepticism has kept the model grounded. Regina Goulding has spent countless hours discussing the model with me, helping to clarify and focus it. Ann Womack's clinical creativity has contributed ideas and techniques from the very beginning, and her pioneering efforts in applying it to medical problems have been inspiring. Working with Rich Simon on various projects has challenged and shaped my thinking and writing, adding clarity and depth; in addition, he generously allowed me to use in this book several excerpts of articles I wrote for the *Family Therapy Networker*. Mike Nichols's advice, editing and support have also been invaluable. My all-too-short time working with Bart Mann was extremely generative, as have been recent discussions with Teresa Jacobson.

Among those who have clarified aspects of the IFS model or pioneered particular applications of it, I wish to recognize Susan Hoke; Annette Hulefeld, Tom Holmes, Paul Ginter, and Nancy Ging; Sharon Pelletier, Barbarra Gould, and Ken Cozzi; Trish Fazzone; Rob Pasick and Nancy Burgoyne; Bob Thorud, Susan Gregory, and the staff of Onarga Academy; Peter Thomas; David Calof; Sandra Watanabe; Dorsey Cartwright; and Joel Van Dyke.

I feel fortunate to have had long-standing relationships with five colleagues who have shaped my thinking, and have also contributed to and supported the development of the IFS model. Doug Breunlin was my partner in our early clinical and intellectual adventures; our collaboration produced the foundation of systemic thought that I later brought to intrapsychic process. In the early 1980s, I learned a great deal from Mary Jo Barrett's insights and courage while we struggled together to understand and treat bulimic clients. With considerable foresight, she pointed out the extremes of thought and behavior that plague these clients. Betty Mac Kune-Karrer aided and abetted the development of the model through her unique multicultural perspective and through providing administrative support that freed me to explore. Howard Liddle provided an early appreciation for structural family therapy and a passion for writing. Doug Sprenkle helped me learn to trust my Self and to think more rigorously.

Let me also thank those who aided editorially. It is wonderful to work with an editor who is excited about what you are trying to do, and at The Guilford Press, Suzanne Little grasped the vision of the book and helped shape it. I am very grateful to Seymour Weingarten, who has been more than patient and supportive while he waited for this. I also received useful comments from Michael Huss, Schlomo Ariel, Ted Schwartz, and Alan Gurman.

Finally, I have been blessed to be surrounded by wonderful families (both of origin and of procreation). Gen Schwartz's love and sensitivity have helped me give the same to my internal and external families. Ted Schwartz instilled an insatiable curiosity and mission of compassion that drive me still. He and Gen created an environment of intellectual stimulation that my five brothers—Steven, Michael, David, Jonny, and Tommy—and I maintain with one another. My daughters, Jessie, Sarah, and Hali, when they're not saying "Get out of here with that parts stuff, Daddy," have been delightfully enchanted with their inner lives and occasionally have let me in on them. Also, they have brought forth parts of me I never knew existed and have learned to love. To my wife, Nancy, I owe the greatest debt. She has tolerated my passion for this model and made sacrifices in my pursuit of it, while also challenging and contributing to it. Over the years our inner protectors have locked horns and hurt each other, but our Selves and many other parts maintain an abiding love. This process has been as healing as it has been educational.

Contents

Journey toward a New Model

> The ways of thinking evolved by psychiatrists in order to
> understand the family as a system will come to be applied in
> understanding the individual as a system. This will be a
> fundamental change within the home territory of psychology . . .
> *—Gregory Bateson (1970, p. 243)*

This book contains new principles and techniques for understanding and changing intrapsychic systems. It also extends these principles and techniques to human systems in general—to families, communities, and countries.

It is the product of a journey that has consumed my life for more than a decade. From my days of astonishment in the early 1980s when my clients began describing inner entities they called parts, through epiphanies of discovery as the operation of internal systems became clearer, this model has held me in its grasp. I remain in awe of the multiplicity phenomenon (the subdivided nature of the mind, to be described further in Chapter 1), and still find each session to be a wonderful adventure as I await the unfolding of the next technique or principle.

Now, however, the adventure is less precarious and more productive. This is because my colleagues, my clients, and I have developed the basic concepts and methods described in this book, which allow this work to be focused, powerful, and yet safe. We have learned the hard way how to enter the intrapsychic realm in a respectful and sensitive way; to help each client differentiate his or her Self, a core of compassion and strength; and to depolarize embattled inner antagonists and help them into preferred, valuable roles. In addition, we have learned how to bring forth these hidden resources to bring harmony and balance to couples and families.

Although the model presented in this book—the internal family systems (IFS) model—is unique and was developed independently of other models, it was not created from whole cloth. It extends the stream of ideas and methods emanating from two different sources: explorations of intrapsychic process and of family process. Part of the model's uniqueness is that it brings these two streams together, creating a confluence that enriches each and also produces something new—a systemic approach to the mind.

As I struggled to construct this model, I learned of others that respected the multiplicity of the mind. Each time I encountered such a model, I had a mixed reaction. On the one hand, I worried that in IFS I had simply rediscovered the wheel; each time, however, I would gradually realize with relief that although there were similarities, the IFS model was indeed a unique advance. The other reaction was a strong sense of confirmation. Here were various therapists or theorists who, independently of one another, had made remarkably similar observations regarding the existence of subpersonalities in all of us. Like me, none of these explorers had preconceptions about multiplicity or set out to create such models. Rather, each was led to this conclusion by listening carefully and openly to clients describing their inner lives.

Trusting Clients

Working with parts of people is neither new nor uncommon. (Indeed, I have learned recently that shamans of various indigenous cultures have been doing similar work for centuries. See Harner, 1990; Ingerman, 1991.) For every therapist, highly qualified teachers in the form of their clients come in and out of the office every day. Thus, it is no surprise that many therapists have been taught to work in creative ways with parts. The goal of this book is to honor and supplement that work, rather than to replace it.

Much of what is contained in this book was taught to me by my clients. Not only did they teach the contents of this approach; they also taught me to listen to them and trust their reports of what happened inside them, rather than to fit their reports into my preconceptions. This lesson was several years in the learning. I had to be corrected repeatedly. Many times clients forced me to discard ideas that had become mainstays of the theory. I also wrestled perpetually with my skeptical parts, which could not believe what I was hearing, and worried about how these reports would be received by academic colleagues. The reason why this model has immediate intuitive appeal for many people is that ultimately I was sometimes able to suspend my preconceptions, tune down my inner skeptics, and genuinely listen.

The history of psychotherapy is rife with examples of times when therapists stopped listening. As Judith Herman (1992) chronicles, Sigmund Freud's early investigations into the etiology of hysteria had this quality of genuine curiosity, as he and others like Pierre Janet spent countless hours interviewing women with hysterical symptoms about their inner lives. "[Freud's] case histories reveal a man possessed of such passionate curiosity that he was willing to overcome his own defensiveness, and willing to listen. What he heard was appalling. Repeatedly his patients told him of sexual assault, abuse, and incest" (Herman, 1992, p. 13). His curiosity led him to the culturally unthinkable. After writing one paper on these findings of sexual trauma, Freud recanted his trauma theory and began generating alternative explanations that did not implicate men; to do this, he had to stop listening and start interpreting. Whereas his early case studies revealed a collaborative relationship with patients, in his last one on hysteria—about the famous Dora, whose father was offering her to his friends as a sexual toy—Freud ignored her outrage and humiliation, and insisted on exploring her erotic feelings as if she desired the situation (Herman, 1992).

As a result of Freud's shift from respectful and curious listening to intellectualized interpreting, psychoanalysis surrounded useful observations about unconscious phenomena (e.g., transference, projection, repetition compulsion, and what can be seen as descriptions of groups of parts—the id, ego, and superego) with convoluted explanations that were removed from people's experience (e.g., penis envy, wish fulfillment, drive theory). Freud influenced generations of theorists to trust their theories more than their clients.

Carl Gustav Jung was able to listen only after he broke with Freud. Because he had no theory to hold onto for security, he had to reach out to his patients for help:

> After the parting of the ways with Freud, a period of inner uncertainty began for me. It would be no exaggeration to call it a state of disorientation. I felt totally suspended in mid-air, for I had not yet found my own footing. Above all, I felt it necessary to develop a new attitude toward my patients. I resolved for the present not to bring any theoretical premises to bear upon them, but to wait and see what they would tell of their own accord. (1962, p. 165)

Only recently have therapists begun emerging from the cloud of arcane theory and listening once again. Again, they are hearing about sexual abuse and other forms of trauma. They are also hearing about parts.

Explorers of Inner Space

Some therapists/theorists listened to their clients and consequently walked segments of this intriguing inner road before me. They provided lanterns and maps for some of the territory, while for other stretches I have had only my clients as guides. For the first few years after entering this intrapsychic realm, I assiduously avoided reading the reports of others, for fear that my observations would be biased by preconceptions of what existed and was possible. Gradually I felt secure enough to compare my observations with others who had directly interacted with inner entities. I was astounded by the similarity of many observations, yet intrigued by some of the differences. I mention some of the strongest influences below.

The Italian psychiatrist Roberto Assagioli (1973, 1965/1975) is credited by some as the first Western thinker to discover the multiplicity of the mind. Originally a champion of Freud's psychoanalysis, he began writing about subpersonalities in the early 1900s, and his ideas developed into a widespread school of psychotherapy (although it never became part of the mainstream) called psychosynthesis. Reading about psychosynthesis was both amazing and confirming. Here were many of the same things my clients had been telling me about their parts and their Selves. Although followers of psychosynthesis were more interested in helping people get to know individual subpersonalities than in helping them to understand and change the whole internal system, and similarly were more interested in helping people to achieve the full potential of their subpersonalities than in helping them to solve problems and heal syndromes, reading about psychosynthesis strengthened the conviction that I was on the right track and provided new directions.

Jung was 13 years older than and was acquainted with Assagioli, and remains the best-known advocate of multiplicity. Much of Jung's knowledge of inner beings was direct: In middle age, he began to journey inside himself. Whereas Assagioli saw a variety of subpersonalities, Jung classified these entities into complexes, which are generally negative, and archetypes, which are generally positive. He also used such terms as the persona, the shadow, the animus, and the anima to describe them further. Jung's (1962, 1968, 1969) conceptualization of multiplicity was further removed than Assagioli's from my observations because of his tendency to presuppose the nature of these inner inhabitants, based on their derivation from a collective unconscious. He developed a technique of direct interaction with parts called active imagination (Hannah, 1981), however, which is related to the method called in-sight and described in Chapters 4 and 5 of this book.

Both Jung and Assagioli subscribed to the idea that, in addition to subpersonalities, each person contains a Self or Center that is different from the parts. As both saw it, this Self is a state of mind to be achieved—a place of nonjudgmental, clear perspective (although Jung also discussed Self as the total personality at times). According to Jung, this Self is a passive, observing state. According to Assagioli, a person can eventually evolve to a point at which the Self shifts from passive observer to active manager of the personality.

Before I learned of these conceptions, many clients had described having such a core Self to me. We had experimented with letting their Self lead as soon as possible in the process of working with their parts. Through the application of family therapy techniques, I had stumbled onto ways to help people quickly find and actively use these resources. Reading of a comparable, if less active, Self in the models of Jung and Assagioli was confirming, and also left me excited at the prospect that no one had fully explored the potential of Self-leadership.

I went on to read the work of Jungian authors who had refined the active imagination process (Hillman, 1975; Johnson, 1986), as well as that of other Jungians who had developed an approach called voice dialogue for interacting with what they termed inner voices and for getting to know the Self (Stone & Winkelman, 1985). At the same time I had several stimulating encounters with Sandra Watanabe, a local therapist who had developed a method resembling voice dialogue for working with what she called internal characters (Watanabe, 1986). I also became acquainted with the work of others who seemed to be on similar paths (Beahrs, 1982; J. Watkins, 1978; M. Watkins, 1986), or, as in the case of Gestalt therapy's open-chair technique (Perls, 1969), had developed methods for accessing and working with multiplicity (see also Bandler & Grinder, 1982). While exploring all these sources, I tried to let my clients and their parts decide which concepts or methods seemed most valid or useful.

Reading this literature also crystallized a major difference between myself and these explorers. By and large, these theorists thought about and treated subpersonalities individually; they encouraged clients to get to know their parts one at a time. There was little written about the relationships that parts formed with one another, about the way a whole intrapsychic system operated, or about the way a person's intrapsychic system compared to his or her family system. Similarly, most of the techniques for working with subpersonalities were individually based. Ways of treating a group of parts as a system or inner family had not been fully explored. It was that gap that I attempted to use my family therapy training to fill.

Family Therapy

Born in part as a reaction against the acontextual excesses of the psychoanalytic movement, the systems-based models of family therapy traditionally eschewed issues of intrapsychic process. It was assumed that the family level is the most important system level to change, and that changes at this level trickle down to each family member's inner life. Although this taboo against intrapsychic considerations delayed the emergence of more comprehensive systemic models, the taboo had the beneficial effect of allowing theorists to concentrate on one level of human system until useful adaptations of systems thinking could evolve.

I was one of these "external-only" family therapists for the first 8 years of my professional life. I obtained a PhD in marital and family therapy, so as to become totally immersed in the systems thinking that I found so fascinating and valuable. I was drawn particularly to the structural school of family therapy (Minuchin, 1974; Minuchin & Fishman, 1981), largely because of its optimistic philosophy. Salvador Minuchin asserted that people are basically competent but that this competence is constrained by their family structure; to release the competence, change the structure. The IFS model still holds this basic philosophy, but suggests that it is not just the external family structure that constrains and can change. In addition, the IFS overlays some structural methods, particularly the boundary-making technique, on internal family process.

From the strategic school of family therapy (Haley, 1976; Watzlawick, Weakland, & Fisch, 1974), I learned the importance of tracking and understanding sequences of interaction. The positive feedback loop, known also as the more-of-the-same sequence or the vicious circle, remains a centerpiece of my systems thinking. An example of such a sequence is when family member A tries to change family member B, who reacts by becoming more extreme. A then tries more of the original attempted solution, which further activates B, resulting in a rigid, polarized relationship.

Jay Haley (1980) expanded the focus on sequences to include longer circular sequences that play out over months or decades in families. Cloe Madanes (1981) emphasized the protective role that symptomatic family members play—a notion that has helped in understanding the protective roles internal personalities are often forced to adopt. In addition, the hypnotherapist Milton Erickson, who strongly influenced the strategic school, was one of the first to hold the conviction that the unconscious is a source of wisdom and strength rather than a repository of interfering drives.

Some of Murray Bowen's (1978) ideas have also been influential and parallel some IFS concepts. His concept of "differentiation of self" is quite similar to that of IFS, although the self Bowen would differentiate is perhaps more cerebral than the Self in IFS. His goal of helping people maintain differentiated selves in the presence of family members and sending clients on "family-of-origin voyages" also have parallels within IFS. Bowen also pioneered the study of how families and their problems evolve over many generations. Similarly, the IFS model is concerned with ways in which burdens, in the form of extreme beliefs or feelings, are transferred across generations.

In the 1980s, family therapy underwent a shift in the stance of the therapist—from the highly interventive and directive one of the structural and strategic schools to a more collaborative position. Some advocates of the Milan model of family therapy (Selvini Pallazzoli, Boscolo, Cecchin, & Prata, 1978) were at the vanguard of this shift and influenced therapists to take a stance of genuine curiosity toward families (Cecchin, 1987). This movement generated a style of interviewing called "circular questioning" (Tomm, 1985, 1987, 1988). The respectful, collaborative stance of the IFS therapist is an extension of this movement.

A more recent influence from the family therapy field has been the work of Michael White of Australia (White, 1989, 1991, 1992; White & Epston, 1990). Like many in the field, he has recently abandoned systems thinking for the narrative metaphor, in which people's lives are seen as governed by the stories they have absorbed about themselves. He helps people find their own stories and deconstruct the stories that have been imposed on them by their families or our culture. This is similar to the process of liberation that people experience when, in IFS therapy, they differentiate their Selves and can examine the stories (burdens) that their parts have accumulated.

Finally, Virginia Satir (1972, 1978a, 1978b) cleared much of the brush along this path of combining the study of intrapsychic subpersonalities with systems theory. To date, she has been the only prominent family therapist to write about parts of people (Satir, 1978a; Satir & Baldwin, 1983). While the others were caught up in the cold, detached world of mechanistic systems thinking, she listened to her heart and, in the face of disdain from the field, remained on this path of increasing self-esteem through self-awareness. Since during my formative years I was one of those who saw her work as too "touchy/feely," my admiration for her trailblazing approach has come later, particularly as I encounter similar criticisms.

The distillation of these influences from family therapy can also be found in the book *Metaframeworks: Transcending the Models of Family Therapy* (Breunlin, Schwartz, & Mac Kune-Karrer, 1992). In it, Doug Breunlin, Betty Mac Kune-Karrer, and I have culled useful elements of the different schools of family therapy into a series of six conceptual frameworks that are interconnected by common presuppositions. The IFS model is one of these frameworks, which also include organization, sequences, development, gender, and culture. In a way, the present book is an expansion of some of the ideas outlined in *Metaframeworks*, but with IFS as the overarching framework.

CHAPTER 1

The Basic Concepts: Multiplicity and Systems

I looked at my father with warm gratitude. His feedback and encouragement over the past year had enriched my book, which now was almost done. I told him excitedly, "I finally figured out how to begin the book. I'll start with a personal anecdote." My father looked at me from behind his newspaper and said, "That sounds good," in a flat, distracted tone. I felt a surge of resentment slide up from my gut, making my face flush and my head throb. Suddenly the affection and excitement I had been enjoying disappeared. "He just doesn't care about my work," I thought. "He never cared about my ideas or about me." I looked again at my father's face, and it seemed harder, more angular. Somewhere inside I had a vague sense that I was overreacting, but this didn't stop me from storming out of the room, vowing to myself never again to talk to my father about the book.

What happened here? Did I simply lose my temper (what does "losing one's temper" mean, exactly)? In a sense, I changed temporarily into a very different person, complete with different feelings and thoughts, but also different ways of sensing and seeing the world and of moving and talking. Indeed, my father literally looked different to me after the shift—more menacing and less sympathetic. What became of the person I was before the shift? Did the tidal wave of resentment wash that person away or simply cover him over? Who then am I? Am I the resentful person or the affectionate one, or both? Or am I the one who knew I was overreacting, or someone entirely different?

What are we to make of what seem to be different personalities within people? Are they merely sets of cognitions and emotions, or are they something more? How did they develop? How do they relate to one another and to other people? How are they affected by the person's past, family, or culture? How can they change?

These are fundamental questions with which philosophers have grappled over the millenia, but with which psychologists have struggled especially intensely in the 20th century. The answers have determined the way people relate to one another and to their problems. Because they shape our civilization, these answers are extremely important. This book contains a fresh set of answers, derived in large part from the guidance of clients themselves.

The goal of this book is to introduce a new way of thinking about and changing the human condition, called the internal family systems (IFS) model. Although some elements of IFS are similar to elements of other models and will seem familiar to many readers, IFS represents a new synthesis of two paradigms. One of these is called the multiplicity of the mind—the idea that we all contain many different beings. The other is known as systems thinking. Each of these paradigms has been available for decades, but never before have they been combined. Combining them produces a model of psychotherapy that has many valuable qualities.

For example, by viewing intrapsychic process as a system, the IFS model allows therapists to relate to every level of human system—intrapsychic, familial, community, cultural, societal—with the same concepts and methods. These concepts and methods are ecologically sensitive, in that they focus on understanding and respecting the network of relationships among the members of human systems at any level. This ecological approach allows people to minimize the distress to their systems as they change and to make informed decisions regarding the value and timing of change attempts.

The IFS model also produces a form of psychotherapy that is collaborative, nonpathologizing, and enjoyable. It is nonpathologizing in that people are viewed as having all the resources they need, rather than as having a disease or deficit. Instead of lacking resources, people are seen as being constrained from using innate strengths by polarized relationships both within themselves and with the people around them. The model is designed to help people release these constraints, thereby releasing their resources.

Moreover, because people already have the resources they need, therapists can collaborate with them rather than teaching them, confronting them, or trying to fill putative holes in their psyches or families. The approach is enjoyable for therapists, because it relieves them of sole responsibility for directing and controlling the course of therapy and for making key interpretations or directives. Instead, direction and discovery emerge spontaneously as clients get to know themselves and one another. It also takes therapists on fascinating journeys into their clients' (and their own) inner and outer worlds, expanding options and releasing resources at every level.

It should be emphasized at this point that to use this model effectively, the reader does not have to adopt the total package of concepts and methods. Many of the IFS principles and techniques can be incorporated into other models with which the reader is more comfortable or familiar. Indeed, it is a mistake to overidentify the IFS model with the group of techniques presented in Chapters 4 and 5. Any number of techniques can be used to access the multiplicity phenomenon, and those emphasized in this book are merely those with which I am most comfortable and familiar. Just as family therapy is not a set of techniques for working with the family group, but rather is a way of viewing people as embedded in the context of their relationships, so the IFS model is a new way of understanding people that informs a rich variety of methods. Rather than a collection of techniques, then, the IFS model is the collection of principles described here.

To illustrate the IFS model, I have drawn many of the examples from my experience with bulimic clients and their families. I have been fascinated by bulimia for over a decade and have learned much of what is in this book from these clients. In addition, one cannot study bulimia without being struck by the parallels among the conflicts within these individuals (primarily young women), within their families, within various cultures, and within our society. Few other problems make these internal and external parallels more obvious and easily understood. Finally, there is a universality to bulimic clients' predicaments. We all have been hurt in life and have used various methods to escape or soothe that pain. We all must relate to food, and we all, at least at times, have related to food in extreme ways.

Although many of the examples in this book involve bulimia, the IFS approach has been useful with the full range of clinical problems. My colleagues, my trainees, and I use the model as our basic orientation to human systems. Consequently, we apply aspects of the model in all our psychotherapy and with a wide variety of issues or syndromes. The question of whether there are types of problems for which the model is contraindicated is a complex one, which is discussed in more detail in Chapter 9. Suffice it to say here that because IFS is a basic orientation to people, it becomes impossible not to use the model, at least at the level of how one understands people and their problems. Also, there are many different levels of applying the model—from simply using the parts language at one end of a continuum, to accompanying a person on a journey into his or her intrapsychic world at the other. So a therapist can tailor the level of method to the severity or delicateness of the problem.

Although this book offers a systemic view of intrapsychic process, its scope is wider. The IFS principles are applicable to family, and cultural, and societal levels as well. If the reader becomes fascinated with the parallels that exist across human systems, then the book will have succeeded.

It will also succeed if the reader becomes intrigued by the multiplicity phenomenon and is encouraged to try the IFS approach, but is careful to heed the book's warnings and follow its guidelines. The IFS model of treatment has evolved gradually yet dramatically over the past decade. It is only in the last several years that my colleagues and I feel confident that we have identified and successfully addressed key obstacles to using the model safely in general practice.

Multiplicity of Mind

Most of us have been socialized to believe that a person has one mind. We are taught that though a person has disparate thoughts and feelings, they all emanate from a unitary personality. As Hermann Hesse lamented, "it appears to be an inborn and imperative need for all men to regard the self as a unit. However often and however grievously this illusion is shattered, it always mends again" (Hesse, 1927/1975, p.). As a result, most people have a poor self-concept because they believe that the many extreme thoughts and feelings they experience constitute who they are. As Elizabeth O'Connor (1971) writes, "If I say 'I am jealous,' it describes the whole of me, and I am overwhelmed by its implications. The completeness of the statement makes me feel contemptuous of myself."

This view of the personality as unitary leads to all manner of unnecessary despair. For example, when Bill's anger covers over his affection for his wife, Mary, he panics because he believes *he* no longer loves her. When he feels incompetent and hopeless, he is paralyzed, believing that is who he really is. When, in the midst of a fight, Mary says, "I hate you," Bill thinks even after her postfight apologies that she really does hate him deep down, because "*she* wouldn't have said it if *she* didn't mean it."

Although we have psychological theories that describe humans complexly, in practice our mental health system also tends to operate on this monolithic basis. Our diagnostic categories have come to be used as descriptions of a person's one personality. It is not uncommon to hear therapists say they are treating a "borderline" or a "depressive" or some other label, as if such a label encapsulates a client's character. We focus on a person's most extreme feelings or thoughts and consider them to be their most basic ones—manifestations of their essential, defective nature.

This monolithic thinking permeates our culture despite the many models of the mind that subscribe to some degree of multiplicity. Freud brought to light the disturbing fact that there are hidden, mysterious elements of personality that communicate symbolically. He brought the existence of an intrapsychic closet out of the closet, so to speak. How strange it must have been to think that unconscious components of the psyche keep things from the rational, managerial mind with which people identify! Freud (1923/1961) opened the door for exploration of multiplicity with his descriptions of the id, ego, and superego. Various post-Freudian theorists have moved beyond his tripartite model and discussed a range of inner entities. Perhaps the most influential of these is object relations theory, which, since Melanie Klein in the 1940s, has asserted that our internal experience is shaped by introjected "objects," holograph-like representations of significant people in our lives (Klein, 1948; Gunthrip, 1971).

Jung (1935/1968, 1963, 1968, 1969), in his discussion of archetypes and complexes, took the notion that we contain many minds a step further, because he considered them as more than just introjects. In 1935, Jung (1935/1968) described a complex as having the

> tendency to form a little personality of itself. It has a sort of body, a certain amount of its own physiology. It can upset the stomach, it upsets the breathing, it disturbs the heart—in short, it behaves like a partial personality. . . . I hold that our personal unconscious, as well as the collective unconscious, consists of an indefinite, because unknown, number of complexes or fragmentary personalities. (pp. 80–81)

Jung's younger contemporary Roberto Assagioli (1973, 1965/1975; Ferrucci, 1982) also posited that we are a collection of subpersonalities, as I have noted in the Introduction. Since Assagioli, a large number of theorists have recognized our natural multiplicity; in exploring this territory, they have made observations that are remarkably similar to one another. A more detailed history of the recognition of multiplicity is available in the book *Subpersonalities* (Rowan, 1990), and a list of references on approaches that subscribe to the multiplicity of the mind is provided in Appendix C of the present book.

Regardless of orientation, most theorists who have explored intrapsychic process have described the mind as having some degree of multiplicity. Scanning the currently influential psychotherapies, we find that object relations describes internal objects (Klein, 1948; Gunthrip, 1971; Fairbairn, 1952; Kernberg, 1976; Winnicott, 1958, 1971); self psychology speaks of grandiose selves versus idealizing selves (Kohut, 1971, 1977); Jungians identify archetypes and complexes (Jung, 1968, 1969); transactional analysis posits many different ego states (Berne, 1961, 1972); Gestalt therapy works with the top dog and underdog (Perls, 1969; Fagan & Sheppard, 1970); and cognitive–behavioral therapists describe a variety of schemata and possible selves (Markus & Nurius, 1987; Dryden & Golden, 1986). Although these theories vary regarding the degree to which the inner entities are viewed as autonomous and possessing a full complement of emotions and cognitions, as opposed to being interdependent, unidimensional, specialized mental units, they all suggest that the mind is far from unitary.

Trauma theory, which undergirds the literature on multiple personality disorder (MPD), views them as fragments of the once unitary personality. Experts on MPD recognize the multiplicity of their patients; however, they view these personalities as the result of early trauma and abuse, which forced the person to split off many "alter" personalities (Kluft, 1985; Bliss, 1986; Putnam, 1989).

Regardless of the theorized source of inner entities (learning, trauma, introjection, the collective unconscious, or the mind's natural state), some of these theorists, more than others, view them as complete personalities. They share a belief that these internal entities are more than clusters of thoughts or feelings, or mere states of mind. Instead, they are seen as distinct personalities, each with a full range of emotion and desire, and of different ages, temperaments, talents, and even genders. These inner people have a large degree of autonomy, in the sense that they think, say, and feel things independent of the person within whom they exist. The MPD theorists hold this view, although they limit it to highly traumatized people. Jung's later writing describes archetypes and complexes in ways that approach autonomous multiplicity, as does a Jungian derivative called voice dialogue (Stone & Winkelman, 1985). In addition, ego state therapy, developed by hypnotherapists John and Helen Watkins (J. Watkins, 1978; J. Watkins & Johnson, 1982; J. Watkins & Watkins, 1979), and Assagioli's psychosynthesis subscribe to full-personality multiplicity.

This is also the position taken in this book. This position—that it is useful to conceive of inner entities as autonomous personalities, as inner people—is contrary to the common-sense notion of ourselves. A person has one body, one brain, so there must only be one being within the person. This is partly why the approaches mentioned above have been viewed as esoteric and remain out of the psychological mainstream. Although anthropomorphizing the subselves may make some readers uncomfortable, and may make it easier for them to relegate the IFS model to the exile of esoterica, it is the way people describe these internal entities (or the entities describe themselves) as people become better acquainted with them. The patterns and characteristics of parts described in this book are not the product of my fevered imagination; they are what clients have reported to me and my colleagues. For this reason, anthropomorphizing is not an appropriate term, because it implies attributing human qualities to things that do not resemble humans.

It was only after several years of working with people's parts that I could consider thinking of them in this multidimensional way, so I understand the difficulty this may create for many readers. In the spirit of curious listening described in the Introduction, however, I respect the full-personality depiction rather than impose a theoretical construct (e.g., schema or internal object) that might be more generally acceptable.

To use the IFS model, one does not have to believe in an ontological sense that parts are internal people. Many therapists view this depiction merely as a useful metaphor and have success with the approach. From a pragmatic perspective, however, the inhabitants of our internal systems respond best to that kind of respect, so it is best to treat them that way—to attribute to them human qualities and responses. Some therapists resolve this problem by not viewing parts as people when they are theorizing, but seeing them as inner people when they are treating clients. I find that dichotomizing my thinking in that way only creates more confusion. This issue is discussed further in Chapter 5.

The notion of inner personalities is becoming less esoteric in U.S. society. It has been popularized recently by the admonition to "heal the injured child within." This message began within the Twelve-Step-addictions movement, and with the help of charismatic leaders like John Bradshaw it has become a national obsession. In this movement, what is meant by the "child within" varies, depending on the writer. Most see it as a metaphor for an innocent state of mind, but some relate to it as a child-like subpersonality. Although no new theory of personality has emerged from this movement, it has helped thousands of people become aware of the existence of different personalities within them.

In addition, the MPD movement, also highly visible across the United States, is helping therapists become more comfortable working with subpersonalities; many such therapists are becoming more open to the idea that their MPD clients are not the only ones who have parts. Indeed, the increasing reports of MPD may be, in part, the result of the increased number of therapists asking clients about their personalities. As clients describe their inner families, some therapists assume that they "have a multiple" on their hands. From the IFS perspective, then, MPD is one way a person's inner family organizes after being chronically and severely hurt. The MPD client's inner family is more polarized, isolated, and protective. Therefore it is less cohesive and more tortured, but otherwise no different from the inner families of people who have not been hurt so badly.

Thus, our culture seems to be gradually warming to the idea of multiplicity. Another sign of this is that the postmodernist movement, which is having a powerful influence in virtually all the social sciences, has rejected the idea of a unitary self. Instead, many postmodern writers celebrate multiplicity, extolling the virtues of a self that contains a plurality of disparate personalities, just as they advocate a pluralistic view of society. For example, the French feminist Hélène Cixous (1974, p. 397) writes: "Understand it the way it is: always more than one, diverse, capable of being all those it will at one time be, a group acting together, a collection of singular beings that produce the enunciation. Being several and insubordinable, the subject can resist subjugation." Sandra Harding (1986, p. 247) echoes this view: "I argue for the primacy of fragmented identities . . . within a unified opposition, a solidarity against the culturally dominant forces of unitarianism." Pluralism involves an attempt to hold unity and diversity in balance, to value the many within the one, to resolve conflict without imposing synthesis or expelling groups, and to celebrate difference. Multiplicity of the mind involves this kind of pluralism.

Most postmodernists go no further in their statements about the self because of their general aversion to the kind of grand theories and intrapsychic pronouncements they believe have characterized modernism. In the sense that the IFS model is a large-scale theory that explores intrapsychic process, it swims against the postmodernist intellectual current. As a result, it will be ignored by some postmodernist thinkers even if they are attracted to its celebration of multiplicity.

In addition to this evolution within psychotherapy and society, there are parallel shifts toward a multiplicity-based view of the mind within the fields of artificial intelligence and psychoneurology. For example, Michael Gazzaniga is a noted brain researcher whose early studies of the different functions of the right and left hemispheres in the 1950s and 1960s altered our ideas about how thinking occurs. His more recent research has led him to conclude that the original distinction between right- and left-hemisphere function was simplistic. In the book *The Social Brain* (Gazzaniga, 1985), he contends that the human mind actually consists of an undetermined number of independently functioning units he calls modules, each of which has a special role. According to Gazzaniga, our emotional and cognitive lives are shaped by the relationship among our modules. His description of modules and the way they operate is remarkably similar to the IFS conception of parts.

The fields of computer science and artificial intelligence are also converging on a multiplicity-based analogue for the mind. In the original conception of the mind used by computer scientists, the von Neumann model, information was thought to be stored in one area and processed in another. Only one cluster of information was believed to be processed at a time. That is, information was thought to go from one area to another in a serial manner, like an assembly line in a factory.

More recently, researchers have developed parallel processing computers in which many different processors work side by side, communicating with, but remaining largely independent of, one another. These parallel computers are able to "think" in a way that approximates human intelligence much more closely than the earlier serial computers (Wright, 1986). Marvin Minsky (1986), one of the founders of artificial intelligence, concludes:

> For finding good ideas about psychology, the single-agent image has become a grave impediment. To comprehend the human mind is surely one of the hardest tasks any mind can face. The legend of the single Self can only divert us from the target of that inquiry. (p. 51) . . . All this suggests that it can make sense to think there exists, inside your brain, a society of different minds. Like members of a family, the different minds can work together to help each other, each still having its own mental experiences that the others never know about. (p. 290)

Within psychotherapy, there exists some evidence supporting multiplicity that also should be mentioned. John and Helen Watkins (1979) have followed up on the research of Ernest Hilgard (1977, 1979), who described what has come to be known as the "hidden observer" phenomenon. Through hypnosis, Hilgard induced deafness in some subjects; when he asked them to raise a finger if they could hear him at some level, their fingers rose. He repeated the experiment with subjects hypnotically anesthetized to pain, and found that while they could, for example, hold their hands in ice water for long periods, some "part" of them was experiencing the pain despite their apparent lack of reaction. Watkins and Watkins replicated Hilgard's ice water experiment with some of their clients who had been through ego state therapy, but, in addition to asking whether some part was feeling pain, they asked to speak to that part. One or more of the ego states that they had worked with in their clients emerged, often complaining of the pain (J. Watkins & Watkins, 1979).

Thus we may be at the brink of a transformation in the way human beings are understood—a transformation that has far-reaching implications. If we are naturally multiple, then it is possible that our extreme feelings or thoughts are the results of extremes within just small parts of us, rather than evidence of pathology at our cores. The critical or hurtful things that loved ones say about us in arguments may not represent their "real" feelings, but instead may be the opinion of only one or two angry personalities within them, while a silent majority of other personalities may remain loving. Many medical or psychiatric symptoms can be reframed along similar lines. The clusters of symptoms that traditionally result in monolithic psychiatric diagnoses can be seen through the lens of multiplicity as manifestations of the way a person's system of inner personalities has organized to help the person survive. Rather than diagnosing a person's disease, then, a multiplicity-oriented therapist can help the person explore his or her system of inner parts to understand which of them are distressed and why.

Multiplicity transports us from the conception of the human mind as a single unit to seeing it as a system of interacting minds. This shift permits the same systems thinking that has been used to understand families, corporations, cultures, and societies to be applied to the psyche. The mind then becomes just a human system at one level, embedded within the human systems at many other levels. It can be understood with the same systemic principles and changed with the same systemic techniques. Also, we can more easily understand how the various external system levels affect and are affected by the mind when we view them in the context of systems thinking.

The IFS model evolved out of this recognition of the mind's multiplicity and the attempt to understand and change it by using systems thinking. This process had two unexpected outcomes. First, studying internal systems enriched the understanding of human systems in general. For example, the appreciation of the four concepts to be introduced in the next section—balance, harmony, leadership, and development—came from seeing how central they are for internal systems. Second, the application of systems thinking to internal systems led to the development of ways to help people change intrapsychically that seem to be advances over previous approaches.

Systems Thinking

A "system" can be defined as any entity whose parts relate to one another in a pattern. Thus systems include everything from watches to televisions to transit systems. In addition, by this definition, all biological organisms from bacteria to whales are systems. Human systems include everything from an individual's personality to a nation, and also include belief systems (e.g., a set of laws or cultural traditions).

A system is composed of smaller systems (*subsystems*) but is also part of *larger systems,* just as a state contains counties and cities but is also part of a nation. Thus, depending on one's point of view, any entity being examined will be the system-of-focus, a subsystem of the system-of-focus, or the larger system containing the system-of-focus. For example, some chapters in this book focus on the family. In those chapters, the family is the system-of-focus; the family members and their relationships are subsystems; and the family's ethnic community or society is a larger system.

Let me elaborate on these concepts. As a system is being defined here, a pile of auto parts is not a system. Once those parts are assembled in a certain way, those parts become a system that is more than the sum of those parts They become a car. The auto parts relate in a patterned way (i.e., they have a structure) that creates a system for transportation.

A car is not a *cybernetic system,* in that it cannot self-correct; instead, it is dependent on a driver or mechanic for direction or repair. Cybernetic systems can regulate themselves by being sensitive to, and changing according to, feedback from their environment. A car contains some simple cybernetic subsystems—for instance, the car's thermostat or cruise control. These cybernetic subsystems try to maintain a steady state (*homeostasis*), such as a certain range of temperature or speed, while the larger system is in operation.

Cybernetic systems contain sensors that read *feedback* from changes in the car's environment and trigger automatic adaptations to that feedback. The car enters a cold front, and the heat goes on; the car on cruise control starts up a hill, and the accelerator goes down. The increase in heat or in gas is called *negative feedback* from the cybernetic system, because it has the effect of reducing the deviation from the steady state—that is, bringing the system back within the homeostatic range of temperature or speed. *Positive feedback,* then, amplifies deviations (e.g., the accelerator or heat mechanism gets stuck, pushing the speed or heat well past prescribed limits).

A car has clear *boundaries,* in that it is usually easy to define what is part of the car and what is not. These boundaries are not closed, however, because parts can be replaced or added. When a car enters a highway, it becomes "embedded" in a larger system, which it influences and is influenced by. If the car were to stop suddenly in heavy traffic, it would powerfully alter the flow of traffic. Likewise, the car's speed and ability to maneuver are constrained by the pace of the cars around it. When the highway is less congested, the car is less constrained by (less embedded in) its larger system. Thus, there are degrees to which systems affect one another—degrees to which they are embedded within or constrained by one another.

Now let us look at human systems. All of the concepts outlined above apply to human systems: structure, boundaries, positive and negative feedback, homeostasis, and degrees of embeddedness or constraint. Human systems are certainly cybernetic. People are organized to maintain a range of homeostasis in any number of areas, from proximity to other people to levels of conflict with others. In addition, each person contains a multitude of cybernetic subsystems, from those regulating blood sugar levels to those regulating the expression of feelings. Family therapy borrowed these principles from the study of mechanical or biological systems to try to understand families. Yet people are not merely reactors to environmental feedback. These cybernetic principles are not enough; they are necessary but not sufficient. A human systems perspective needs to include other principles derived from the study of living systems.

Human systems are different in an important way from mechanical systems, and this difference is at the core of the IFS model. A basic premise of IFS is that people have an innate drive toward and wisdom about their own health. They not only try to maintain steady states and react to feedback; they also strive toward creativity and intimacy. They come fully equipped to lead harmonious internal and external lives. From that basic premise, it follows that when people have chronic problems, these inner resources and wisdom are not being fully accessed. Elements in the systems in which they are embedded or that are embedded within them are constraining their access to these resources. IFS therapy is designed to help people find and release these constraints.

Systems thinking helps us examine the various systems surrounding or within a client to find and release constraints. Constraints may exist in a client's system of inner personalities; in the client's relationship with various family members; in the way the family in general is organized; in the way various institutions outside the family affect it (school, work, mental health system, etc.); and in the way the client's ethnic community and the larger society affect the family's values and beliefs. All of these human systems are interlocked. They affect and are affected by one another.

Trying to understand and assess all these levels of human systems would be an overwhelmingly complex task, except that each level operates in similar ways. Outlined below are four key principles of human systems that are not included in the preceding discussion of cybernetic systems: balance, harmony, leadership, and development. These principles have evolved from my work with internal and family systems, but they seem to have some universality. They are discussed in greater detail in Chapters 4 and 6.

1. *Balance*. Human systems function best when they are balanced. What does that mean? What are the qualities that, when out of balance, create problems? I believe that there are four dimensions for which balance is crucial to a system's health: the degree of influence a person or group has on the system's decision making; the degree of access a person or group has to the system's resources; the level of responsibility that a person or group has within the system; and the degree to which the system's boundaries are balanced. In a balanced system, then, each person is allowed the degree of influence, access to the system's resources, and responsibilities appropriate to his or her needs and role in the system,

and equal to those of people in similar roles. In addition, the boundaries defining who can participate in subsystems within the system and how they can participate are neither too rigid nor too diffuse.

2. *Harmony.* The concept of harmony applies to the relationships among people in the system. In harmonious systems, an effort is made to find the role each member desires and for which he or she is best suited. People work cooperatively toward a common vision, yet value and support individual differences in style and vision. That is, the system allows each individual to find and pursue his or her own vision, while trying to fit that individual vision into the larger vision for the system. In such an atmosphere, people do not mind sacrificing some of their personal resources and goals for the greater good. They feel valued for their personal qualities as well as for their contribution, and they care about one another's well-being. They communicate well, in that they are sensitive and responsive to information flowing among the members of the system. The flow of information among members within a system will be called *feedwithin* in this book, to distinguish it from information exchanged with the system's environment, called feedback.

The opposite of harmony is *polarization.* In a polarized relationship, each person in the relationship shifts from a flexible, harmonious position to a rigid, extreme position that is the opposite of or competitive with that of the other. Later I discuss the many ways in which polarizations constrain systems.

3. *Leadership.* Balance and harmony in human systems require effective leadership. One or more members of a system must have the ability and respect to do the following: mediate polarizations and facilitate the flow of feedwithin; ensure that all members are protected and cared for, and that they feel valued and encouraged to pursue their individual vision within the limits of the system's needs; allocate resources, responsibilities, and influence fairly; provide a broad perspective and vision for the whole system; represent the system in interaction with other systems; and honestly interpret feedback from other systems. Fortunately, as I have mentioned earlier, human systems have the resources necessary for this kind of leadership. Those resources are often constrained, however, by a variety of factors to be discussed later.

4. *Development.* Despite being born with the resources necessary for balanced and harmonious living, human systems need time for those resources to develop. An analogy to a new basketball team can be drawn: The team members possess plenty of raw talent, but until they learn one another's habits and come to trust and respect the coach, they will not function optimally. Comparably, the wisdom for health exists within a human system, but it takes time to develop the skills or the relationships necessary to implement that wisdom. Thus, effective leadership and clear

boundaries evolve gradually and are affected by the system's environment. If the system-of-focus is embedded in a harmonious, balanced larger system, then it is likely to have the freedom and support it needs to become harmonious and balanced. A human system's ability to use its resources for healthy development will be constrained, however, if it evolves within a polarized, unbalanced larger system, in which case it will take on the extreme beliefs and emotions of the larger system.

A developing system will also be constrained if it accumulates burdens along the way. This happens when the system is traumatized (thrown out of balance) before it has fully developed. Trauma also has the effect of freezing or fixating members of the system at the point in time of the trauma. These frozen members not only are no longer available to help, but their extreme emotions further constrain the system and force other members into hyperprotective roles.

With these four principles—balance, harmony, leadership, and development—one can assess a human system at any level, as well as the systems containing it or contained within it. If a human system is having problems, one can work with the members of the system to find and release whatever is constraining the system's resources, whether the constraints are imbalances, polarizations, leadership problems, or burdened development. Thus, the IFS model is a constraint-releasing approach. Chapters 4 and 5 elaborate on the common constraints one finds within each of these four principles.

The Example of Bulimia

My colleagues and I began working with bulimic clients and their families in the early 1980s, before much was known about its etiology or treatment. My first encounter with the syndrome occurred, in fact, before I had heard of it. I sat slack-jawed, trying to contain my astonishment as my teenage client shamefully confessed to bouts in which she frantically ate anything she could get her hands on in her parents' house and later vomited all this into the toilet. She said she hated herself for doing it but couldn't stop. She felt out of control—not only of her eating, but also of feelings of the loneliness and rage that seemed to alternate in overwhelming her. She desperately wanted help.

I felt at once confused, intrigued, and overwhelmed. Why would anyone do such a strange thing—stuff oneself only to throw up minutes later? That session was the beginning of a journey that has transformed my views of people, therapy, and U.S. society. In trying to make sense out of what at first seemed to be such bizarre behavior, I was forced to examine all levels of my clients' context, from their internal lives to their families and their cultures. In the process, I discarded many cherished beliefs about people and therapy in favor of the beliefs that make up the IFS approach, as I have described in the Introduction.

In the years since that first session, bulimia has risen from psychiatric obscurity to become a widely discussed and practiced syndrome. In addition to generating a large professional literature, bulimia has become a household word. Countless people (primarily young women) have become slaves to the practice of compulsive binge eating followed by some form of purging—vomiting, ingestion of laxatives or diuretics, obsessive exercise, or fasting. The apparently illogical nature of this behavior, and the meteoric rise in awareness of (and, in all likelihood, incidence of) bulimia, evoke images of a medieval curse upon the land. As the exasperated brother of a client exclaimed in a family session, "What's going on? Six weeks ago I learned about my sister, and now this week my girlfriend tells me she's been doing it for a year. They're everywhere!"

What *is* going on? It is clear that there are many women and some men whose lives are centered around these eating habits, although not as many as 20% of college-age women (the exaggerated figure often cited in the mass media). The more reliable estimates of between 1% and 2% of any group of young women (Fairburn, Hay, & Welch, 1993) still represent an enormous amount of suffering. This syndrome does produce a great deal of suffering, even though its painful aspects are often glossed over. The gluttonous extravagance of the binge and the repulsive aspects of the purge allow people to take bulimia lightly or make jokes about it. These aberrant qualities also contribute to the shame, self-loathing, and embarrassment of bulimic clients, and to the impatience of families and friends.

U.S. society in general, and the dominant or mainstream culture within this society in particular, have little sympathy for those who seem to lack will power; this is especially true regarding what people do with food. Whereas the excessive will power of anorexics sometimes engenders a grudging respect or envy in the people around them the excesses of bulimics are often seen as reflecting a pitiful or disdainful weakness of character. The popular media often take a "scared straight" approach by emphasizing the potential damage to the body inherent in bulimic practices. Often these scare tactics add a layer of fear to the shame that clients already feel, and intensify the urgency and frustration of those around them.

This is not to downplay the real medical dangers associated with bulimia, but to underscore the predicament that bulimic clients and their families are in. The clients want desperately to stop but cannot, and so feel weak and worthless, believing that they are harming themselves while disappointing others. Family members alternate between anger and revulsion at the client's lack of will power, frustration at their inability to help the clients, guilt or recrimination over having caused the syndrome, and fear that the clients are damaging themselves permanently. Solutions are not easily found in such a polarized emotional climate, and therapists can easily be caught up in the polarization. To be helpful, therapists need an approach that depolarizes and empowers these clients and their families.

Some approaches to bulimia have disempowered clients by giving them a pathological diagnosis or seeing them as victims of their families or their cultures. Similarly, family members sometimes have been blamed for inept parenting or for needing clients' symptoms to distract from their own problems or to reassure them that the clients will not grow up and leave them. Although some cases may present evidence for these assumptions, therapists who dwell on this evidence will have trouble maintaining and conveying respect for the resources of the clients and their families, and empathy for the predicament of each. Often a therapist is working with an individual and family members who are heavily constrained by systems within and without. The therapist needs an approach that helps find and release those constraints, rather than one that contributes to the constraints.

When I began working with bulimic clients, I was a young, dyed-in-the-wool structural/strategic family therapist. I believed that the family level was the most influential system level, and that family members needed the bulimics' symptoms as a distractive focus. These assumptions led to several negative consequences. I underestimated my clients' abilities to change themselves. I became a pathology detective with families, trying to sniff out the "real" problems that the bulimia was reflecting or distracting from. I also downplayed the role of cultural pressures on women regarding their appearance, or the role of women's subordinate status in our society. Thus, I overfocused on one level (the family level) of the many levels of systems in which the syndrome of bulimia is embedded; within that level, I overfocused on families' flaws rather than their strengths.

My colleagues and I (R. C. Schwartz, Barrett, & Saba, 1985) reported that many bulimic families resembled the "psychosomatic families" described by Minuchin, Rosman, and Baker (1978), in that they demonstrated the characteristics of enmeshment, overprotectiveness, rigidity, and lack of conflict resolution. In addition, we found these families to be highly isolated, to be acutely conscious of appearances, and to attribute special meaning to food and eating. Root, Fallon, and Friedrich (1986) categorized bulimic families as either perfectionistic, overprotective, or chaotic, depending on the way the families handled such things as conflict or child rearing. My colleagues and I, as well as Root et al., advocated that the treatment of bulimic clients include significant others, whose active participation was seen as crucial to a positive outcome.

The most common approach to treating bulimics, however, has focused on some aspect of individual clients' struggle with themselves. Most of the literature in this area has come from the cognitive–behavioral school, which attempts to change both the behaviors and irrational cognitions that surround binge–purge episodes, whether in group or in individual therapy (see, e.g., Fairburn, Marcus, & Wilson, 1993). More traditional psychodynamic formulations have also been proposed, and it is my impression that although models such as object relations have not dominated the literature, more bulimic clients are treated psychodynamically than any other way because of the general popularity of these models (Johnson, 1991; H. Schwartz, 1986; Swift & Letven, 1984).

Finally, psychopharmacological approaches, which also locate the problem within the individual, have gained momentum on the basis of some outcome studies (see Walsh, 1992, for a review). These theorists tend to downplay the impact of systems at any level other than the physiological.

As is apparent from this brief review, I was part of this montage of disconnected approaches in my emphasis on the importance of family factors over the other levels. One reason why we tunnel-visioned, if not blind, men and women were reporting on only one part of the elephant is that we each had different sets of preconceptions about what the whole animal should look like. The field of psychotherapy has lacked a model that allows us to shift smoothly across systems at different levels, using the same principles to understand each level. This is not just a dilemma with bulimia; it is true of all psychiatric syndromes. The IFS model attempts to address this dilemma by using systems thinking to understand each level, allowing the parallels and interconnections among levels of human systems to become apparent.

Let me end this introduction to bulimia with a note of caution. It is a mistake to view bulimia—or any other psychiatric syndrome—as a homogeneous problem that can be treated by an algorithmic, step-by-step therapy program. Individuals who compulsively binge and purge come from a wide range of living situations, associated symptoms, and styles of relating to the world. For some the bulimia is the central issue in their lives, while for others it is but one of many major problems. Some seem generally passive and self-conscious, while others seem prone to volcanic explosions at the slightest provocation. Some are terribly ashamed of their symptoms and go to great lengths to hide them from everyone, while others talk openly about their struggles. Many have experienced sexual abuse, but many have not. Finally, there are many individuals for whom bulimia is nothing more than a transient experiment that they have resolved without therapy.

The family systems of bulimic clients are equally heterogeneous. Some clients are heavily embedded in protective or conflictual sequences within their families, such that they are perceived and perceive themselves as pivotal to their families' survival; others have been chronically ignored or neglected by key family members, and are not particularly protective of their families. In some families, other members are involved in addictive problems such as substance abuse or gambling; in still other families, the bulimic clients seem to be the only ones struggling with self-control.

How is a therapist to deal with this variety? If a syndrome cannot always be viewed in one simple way—as protective of someone else in the family, as a distress signal to get needed attention, as the result of childhood sex abuse or of improper parenting at an early age, as a power struggle between the client and the parents, or as an excuse for the client who is afraid to grow up—then how can a therapist know what to do?

When my colleagues and I began our treatment project in 1981, bulimia was a new and exotic syndrome for which there were no family systems explanations or maps. In our anxiety, we seized the frames and techniques developed by structural family therapists for other problems and tried them on each new bulimia case. In several instances this approach worked well, so we leaped to the conclusion that the essential mechanism behind bulimia was the triangulation of the client with the parents. In that sense, we became essentialists; we thought we had found the essence, so we could stop exploring and could use the same formula with each new case. Data that contradicted these assumptions were interpreted as the result of faulty observations or imperfect therapy.

Fortunately, we were involved in a study that required close attention to both the process and outcome of our therapy. As our study progressed, the strain of trying to fit contradictory observations into our narrow model became too great, too Procrustean. We were forced to leave the security and simplicity of our original model and face the anomie that accompanies change. We were also forced to listen carefully to clients when they talked about their experiences and about what was helpful to them. We were forced to discard our expert's mind, full of preconceptions and authority, and adopt what the Buddhists call beginner's mind, which is an open, collaborative state. "In the beginner's mind there are many possibilities; in the expert's mind there are few" (Suzuki, 1970, p. 21). In this sense, our clients have helped us to change as much as or more than we have helped them.

The IFS model was developed in this open, collaborative spirit. It encourages the beginner's mind because, although therapists have some general preconceptions regarding the multiplicity of the mind, clients are the experts on their experiences. The clients describe their subpersonalities and the relationships of these to one another and to family members. Rather than imposing solutions through interpretations or directives, therapists collaborate with clients, respecting their expertise and resources. Because each client is an expert collaborator, a therapist does not need to carry an arsenal of preconceptions regarding the nature of a client's problem or family. The answer to the question posed earlier regarding how a therapist can deal with the absence of simplistic frameworks or formulae is that with increased trust in a client's resources, a therapist does not have to be such an expert.

Thus, the various principles and patterns presented in this book are there to provide guidelines for common clinical situations, but are not to be inscribed in the minds of therapists or imposed on clients. Instead, they should be easily overridden when clients' stories do not fit them. It is far more important for therapists to maintain a collaborative, curious, creative state of mind—what I later describe as Self-leadership—than to carry preordained answers into therapy.

This book, then, is on the IFS model.* Chapters 2 through 5 describe IFS theory and technique as applied to individuals. Chapters 6 and 7 do the same for families. Chapter 8 describes the use of IFS principles to understand cultural groups and the larger society, and Chapter 9 ties up loose ends.

To summarize, the IFS model helps therapists create relationships with clients and their families that are uniting and nonblaming. It gives clients access to constraint-releasing resources, and helps clients understand themselves and other family members in a way that promotes open disclosure, empathy, and respect.

---

*These ideas are elaborated and the operation of internal families in general is illustrated in a forthcoming book by Goulding and Schwartz (in press), on the IFS model with survivors of childhood sexual abuse.

CHAPTER 2

Viewing Individuals as Systems

Do I contradict myself?
Very well then I contradict myself,
(I am large, I contain multitudes.)
—*Walt Whitman (1855/1959, p. 68)*

The Importance of Seeing Individuals as Systems

The IFS model brings systems thinking to the intrapsychic realm. Why is this an important contribution? There are many reasons.

Viewing Parts in Context

The first reason is the idea of viewing a member of a system in context. Family therapy helped clinicians understand that the extreme way some people behave is not necessarily a result of personal pathology, but often relates directly to their family contexts. Similarly, a therapist who encounters a client's subpersonalities can easily misunderstand a part's extreme, destructive presentation as the way the part *is*, rather than as the role it is stuck in. Once the therapist appreciates the system in which the subpersonality is nested—the network of relationships that keeps it extreme—the therapist will relate to the part very differently.

In the novel *Night Secrets* by Thomas Cook (1990), the hero describes his perception of a critical part of him:

> He could feel the evil bubble growing in him, the one that made everything a little emptier than it already was. . . . It drifted toward him from out of nowhere now, as if it no longer needed to be called up by any particular thing, but simply

occupied its place as a steadily darkening presence, filling him with hissing accusations about the way he'd lived his life. There were times when he suspected that everyone must have such a specter, but then he'd see a couple laughing in a restaurant or a father playing with his daughter in the park, or even some solitary old woman contentedly reading a newspaper on her bare cement stoop, and they would strike him as people who'd somehow escaped the grasp of a merciless pursuer, had closed the door and thrown the bolt just in time to leave the shadow breathless in the hall. (pp. 161–162)

This is the way many people come to view parts of themselves: as evil, sinister forces. They may see other parts as repulsively weak or needy, and still others as dirty and shameful. With such views as these, it no wonder that people try desperately to close the door and throw the bolt—to lock these parts away, to put them into exile.

Many bulimic clients contain parts that are harshly critical of their appearance, particularly of their weight. It is easy to assume that this is the essential nature of these parts—that perhaps they are introjected critical parents—if one views them out of context. It is possible instead to learn from such subpersonalities about the other parts with which they are polarized: the ones, for example, that urge the clients to binge-eat, or the rageful or sad ones that take over if the clients ever feel good about themselves. When understood in that context, the brutally critical roles make more sense, and the way to help release the parts from these extreme roles becomes clearer.

Ecological Maps

Second, just as it helps a family therapist to know how families commonly organize, it helps to have maps of internal families. If a therapist is aware of common relationships among a client's network of subpersonalities— that is, common alliances and coalitions and why they are formed—the therapist will be able to intervene planfully and sensitively. The therapist can anticipate an internal system's protective reactions and can time interventions accordingly. The therapist can also anticipate reactions from external systems (family, peers, other intimate relationships) and see how the internal and external levels affect one another. This systemic knowledge provides guidelines for restoring balance, harmony, and effective leadership to an internal family, while striving to minimize distress to it and maximize collaboration with its resources.

New Theory and Technique

Third, just as the application of systems thinking to families led to important new ways to view people and help them change, the same has been true with internal families. Although some of the IFS assumptions and techniques are shared by other approaches, many new assumptions and techniques have emerged from this exploration. In addition, the systemic foundation allows a coherent linkage between theory and technique, so that the model maintains a high degree of internal consistency and comprehensiveness. The connection between theory and practice is very clear.

Liberation and Empowerment

Finally, this enterprise of overlaying systems thinking onto the multiplicity of the mind has resulted in assumptions that are liberating and empowering. People are viewed as already containing the resources they need to lead balanced and harmonious lives. The IFS model helps them find and release the constraints on those resources, at both the internal and external levels.

Evolution of the IFS Model: A Case Illustration

In the Introduction and Chapter 1, I have described in general terms how the IFS model evolved. To give a more specific view of how the model developed, I provide a brief case illustration in this section. In later sections, I outline the basic IFS principles for understanding internal systems.

By the winter of 1983, I had been working with Sally for over a year as a part of an outcome study of the impact of family therapy on clients who had bulimia (R. C. Schwartz et al., 1985). My colleagues and I had been applying our structural/strategic model to these families with success, and Sally's family had also responded well. Sally was an attractive 23-year-old who had entered therapy because her habit of bingeing and vomiting made her feel suicidally depressed. Although clients (primarily women) who binge and purge are far from a homogeneous group, most report a constant internal struggle over their compulsions, the outcome of which determines their self-esteem.

Detriangulation Was Not Enough

In Sally's case, our therapy had helped her give up the role of protecting her father from her mother, and both parents had adapted well to this change. As is true of many bulimic clients, Sally had been highly involved in her parents' relationship. She was her father's confidante and her mother's rival, although she felt quite responsible for and guilty about her mother's unhappiness. It had taken many emotional sessions to uncover this constraining triangle and pry it apart.

Warily, Sally had moved from her parents' home into her own apartment, had found a good job, and was making close friends for the first time. We had weathered several episodes in which the increased intensity of her parents' fights and distress had, like a vacuum cleaner, sucked her back to care for them. Her parents were engaged in marital therapy, and it seemed to me that the whole family system was moving to a new level.

Through all of this change, Sally's bulimic symptoms had waxed and waned. But now that she was "detriangulated" and functioning independently, out of the grip of family crises and loyalties, I expected her to discard this nasty binge–purge habit. After all, it was no longer "needed" by Sally or her family. To my dismay Sally, unaware that she was "cured," continued her bulimic behavior, albeit with less frequency and intensity. She was still bingeing and purging enough to keep her from feeling totally healthy and to keep me, with my outcome-study-oriented mentality, from feeling successful. Sally followed religiously a variety of direct and "paradoxical" tasks I suggested, but they worked only temporarily at best.

The Intimacy–Protectiveness Bind

The focus of Sally's inner turmoil had shifted from her parents to her relations with men, which seemed to gyrate drastically. She shifted quickly from one extreme mood to another as she began dating. For example, she would be elated when she thought a perspective boyfriend liked her; as soon as he moved toward more intimacy, however, she alternated between seeing him as a dangerous oppressor and seeing herself as unlovable and repulsive. She would then passively withdraw from the relationship but feel desperately lonely and needy, believing that she had blown her only chance and that no one would ever care about her.

This sense of neediness coupled with her belief in her own repulsiveness put Sally in a bind. She yearned for love and believed she could not get through life without a man to depend on; however, she was convinced that no one could love her repulsive "real" self and that men would reject her if they got close enough to see it. As a result, she repeated the same pattern of rapidly opening herself up to a man, only to retreat suddenly and confusingly at a certain point.

Bulimia as Lover and Persecutor

These retreats would bring on waves of bulimia. Sally resorted to comestible intimacy, since she feared getting comfort from a man. Food provided a temporary solace, a sense of nurturing or treating herself, a filling of her emptiness. It was a secret indulgence that, though calming, also brought tensions of its own, for she couldn't shake the awareness of the dreaded calories mounting in her stomach. She had long since lost her revulsion toward vomiting, and her purge brought an addicting sense of purification. She had a sense that she had "gotten away with something" and felt a temporary sense of peace, not unlike the state following an orgasm or other biological release.

Sally became increasingly obsessed with her weight, believing that her appearance was the sum total of her assets. She felt at the mercy of feedback from men or from the bathroom scale. If the news was bad, she was more compelled to binge, yet she also felt herself to be a total victim of her bulimia. She believed that if only she could shake it, she wouldn't be so afraid to get close and could finally get the love she yearned for.

Sally's bind is characteristic of many addicted clients. They are in a love–hate relationship with their addiction: They depend on it for intimacy, comfort, and distraction, yet blame it for keeping them from what they want. What they often want is to feel cared for, yet they feel unlovable and so expect and fear rejection. Retreat from relationships triggers bulimia, substance use, or other addictive behavior; this behavior triggers retreat; and so on.

Breaking the Taboo

With my "external-only" family therapy orientation, I was at a loss as to how to help Sally with these binds. It seemed that I was confronting the limitations of my structural/strategic model. Out of frustration, I decided to violate the unwritten rule that governed family therapists who considered themselves systemic: I crossed into intrapsychic territory.

I began discussing with Sally what she experienced just before she went on a binge-and-vomit spree. She described a confusing cacophony of inner "voices" that seemed to carry on intense conversations or arguments in her mind. When I pressed her to differentiate these voices, she found—to her and my surprise—that with relative ease she could identify several voices that regularly held heated debates with one another. One voice was highly critical of everything about her, particularly her appearance. Another defended her against that critical voice and blamed her parents or bulimia for her problems. Another made her feel sad, hopeless, and helpless; still another part "took over" and made her binge. I found her inner life fascinating and, as I asked the same questions of other bulimic clients, remarkably similar to others' inner lives.

Most of my bulimic clients reported that their sense of themselves— their feelings, thoughts, and behavior—could shift suddenly and drastically, as if they were repeatedly possessed by different extreme people. As one client lamented, "I go from being a together professional to a scared, insecure child, to a rageful bitch, to an unfeeling, single-minded eating machine in the course of 10 minutes. I have no idea which of these 'I' really am, but whichever it is, I hate being this way." Asking clients to look more closely inside themselves seemed to have the effect of helping them separate the confusing, cacophonous inner noise into a group of entities they called parts. "This part of me is like a little child, and that part is more mature but rigid." They might not like many of these parts, but somehow identifying them seemed to make them less intimidating or overwhelming. They came to see that only little parts of them felt or thought these extreme things, rather than their core selves.

Asking Questions

Because I had no preconceived conceptual framework for these explorations with Sally, I spent many sessions simply asking her and my other clients about the participants in these inner conversations. What were they like? What did they want? How did they get along with one another? Which ones did the clients like and listen to, and which ones did they hate or fear and ignore? The more I explored these questions, the more their descriptions felt familiar to me as a family therapist—as if I were interviewing one family member about the rest of the family. It seemed that each "voice" had a distinct character, complete with idiosyncratic desires, styles of communication, and temperaments. Moreover, these parts interacted much like conflicted family members, alternately protecting and distracting, allying and battling with one another.

The more I learned about these "internal families" in Sally and my other clients, the more I became intrigued with the question of whether the principles and techniques derived from systems thinking that made working with actual families so understandable and effective could apply to these internal systems. I decided to try to extend these concepts and practices into what systems thinkers had previously considered the impenetrable "black box" of the mind.

The Many in the One

> Which one of the many people who I am, the many inner voices inside of me, will dominate? Who, or how, will I be? Which part of me decides?
>
> –Douglas Hofstadter (1986, p. 782)

The multiplicity view implies that each of us consists of many minds. Sally's "voices" emanated from separate personalities, each of which had some autonomy, in that she was not controlling what they said or did. Even after my initial experiences with the "voices" in bulimic clients, it took me a long time to accept this view of the mind because it is so drastically different from our habitual ways of seeing ourselves, and our language continually conditions us to maintain the monolithic view. We describe clients as "needy," "hostile," "nurturing," or "overinvolved," as if the essence of their personalities could be summed up in one or two words. Once one shifts to this multiplicity paradigm, one chafes at simple descriptions or diagnostic categories of what people think, feel, or are.

Revealing Hidden Conversations

Through the day, we regularly pass from personality to personality. Because of the speed and fluidity of this process for most of us, and the fact that we have such a limited vocabulary for distinguishing among these inner entities, we do not usually attend to the ways in which this inner community conducts its business. When therapists observe client families, it is easy to become absorbed in the content and ignore the interactional process; similarly, we may notice thoughts running through our heads without recognizing that they emerge from a range of recurrent types of conversations that we carry on with ourselves. We are capable of having any number of such dialogues going on at the same time. What is more, we can converse with ourselves in many "languages," some of which take place in a private, idiosyncratic vocabulary of images or body sensations rather than a language of words.

As I have tried to apply these ideas, I have been struck by how quickly and easily most people can become aware of their inner personalities if asked to focus on them. It seems that for many of us, once we get beyond our cultural bias toward viewing ourselves as consistent, unitary individuals, the multiplicity paradigm makes immediate intuitive sense. It also makes sense that since our lives are complex and we have to do and think many things at once, we need many specialized minds operating with a certain amount of autonomy and internal communication to accomplish all of this simultaneous activity.

Multiplicity also provides a useful explanation for many mental phenomena, such as the "spontaneous inspiration" involved in creativity, in which the answers to problems come to us "out of the blue" in the middle of the night. Other examples include the sudden personality changes that we each experience to some degree at times in our lives, but are more pronounced in such instances as religious conversions, drug or alcohol intoxication, suddenly falling in or out of love, or MPD, in which people seem to turn into entirely different personalities. These are not simply matters of shifting sets of emotions or thought patterns; they often represent changes to utterly distinct world views, complete with consistent values, interests, beliefs, and feelings. With the multiplicity paradigm, it is much easier to empathize with the common complaint of bewildered family members that the person with the identified problem sometimes "seems like a totally different person."

Parts

The issue arises as to what to call these internal entities. Depending on the model in use, they have been called subpersonalities, subselves, internal characters, archetypes, complexes, internal objects, ego states, or voices, as noted in Chapter 1. I believe that regardless of the label used in formulating theories, the term used clinically should be the one with which clients are most comfortable. For this reason I have adopted the term *part*, since it is how most people describe their own internal conflicts: "Part of me is afraid, but another part says 'Go for it!'" Although this term is far from ideal, in that it has mechanistic connotations and does not impress those who like "professional" language, it is very useful clinically.

There are some clients who are not comfortable with the term part; in such cases, the reader is encouraged to use whatever term the clients prefer. Out of respect for clients' preferences, I have used terms such as aspect, thought, character, feeling, place, and person. For most of my clients, however, the word part works well.

The Compact Edition of the Oxford English Dictionary (1971) carries an obscure definition of the word part that provides some validation for this usage: "A personal quality or attribute, natural or acquired, esp. of an intellectual kind (as a constituent element of one's mind or character)" (p. 2084). In *Much Ado about Nothing* (1598/1974), Shakespeare has Benedick ask Beatrice, "For which of my bad parts didst thou first fall in love with me?" (V.ii.60–61), and Ben Jonson, in 1598, refers to "A gentleman ... of very excellent good partes." There is also an apt reference in the Bible: "Our bones are dried, and our hope is lost: We are cut off from our parts" (Ezekiel 37:11). Thus, there are honorable precedents.

I use the term parts throughout this book when referring to subpersonalities. A part is not just a temporary emotional state or habitual thought pattern. Instead, it is a discrete and autonomous mental system that has an idiosyncratic range of emotion, style of expression, set of abilities, desires, and view of the world. In other words, it is as if we each contain a society of people, each of whom is at a different age and has different interests, talents, and temperaments. In this sense we are all multiple personalities, although few of us have MPD. From this perspective, people diagnosed as having MPD are those who have been so badly hurt that their parts have become polarized to the point of complete isolation from one another.

Parts as Inner People

Although I use one- or two-word labels to refer to individual parts throughout this book (e.g., the Striver, the Evaluator, the Asserter, the Caretaker, the Passive Pessimist, etc.), it is a mistake to overidentify a part with its label. For example, just because Sally's Striver said it wanted her to achieve and had taken the role of pushing her to do so (see below), this did not mean that it was *essentially* a striving part. Instead, I find it best to conceive of such a part as if it were a person who has been forced into a striving role. As a person, however, it has many other feelings and abilities that are not captured by the Striver label and may be better suited for a very different role. The same is true for other parts. For example, a part that is angry may also feel hurt or scared, but if one sees it as "*the* angry part," one is likely to ignore these other feelings and focus exclusively on its assertive role. If, on the other hand, it is viewed as an angry person (often a child or teenager), then one is interested in its other feelings and in helping it discover its preferred role.

Once again, the analogy to a family may make this clear. In many traumatized families, children are forced into extreme roles that they neither want nor are suited for, but believe are necessary for their own and their families' survival. In alcoholic families, for example, one often finds the overresponsible child, the distracter, the angry rebel, the hero, and so forth. These children are forced into these roles by their family dynamics; once released from the roles, they change dramatically and are able to discover what they are really like. An identical process takes place in internal families.

Differences from Other Models

Not surprisingly, all the models of psychotherapy that subscribe to a multiplicity paradigm contain similarities to one another and to the IFS model. The IFS model differs from the others, however, in several ways. First, its focus is not just on a person's individual parts, but also on the networks of relationships among these parts. That is, it attempts to understand and work with the entire internal system. Second, it differs in its emphasis on the connections between "external" (e.g., family, cultural) systems and internal systems, and its ability to use the same concepts and techniques at both levels. Finally, it differs in its assumptions about the qualities and role of what is called the Self.

The Self

As soon as you trust yourself, you will know how to live.
–Johann Wolfgang von Goethe

Is a person simply a collection of parts, or is there something more at the seat of the soul? Initially I believed the former, because I was relying on my clients' descriptions, and all they described were the parts. For instance, I would listen to Sally tell of her relationship with each part—how she felt toward it, how much she listened to it, how much she could control it, how she thought it felt toward her—and I began to wonder who was articulating this. Who was the reporter who was seeing or hearing a part, experiencing its feelings, and describing all this to me? Was it just another part, or was there someone else in there?

Boundary Making

As I began asking clients to interact with their parts in my presence—at first through the Gestalt therapy open-chair technique, and later through imagery—I found that a conversation might be going well until at a certain point the client would become upset with the part and change his or her view of it entirely. Or the person might have extreme feelings toward or beliefs about the part from the outset. I remembered from my work with families that when an interaction between two family members was not going well, it was often because a third family member was interfering—interjecting comments, taking sides, making faces, or in general violating the boundary around the other two family members. The technique of "boundary making" was developed by structural family therapists (Minuchin & Fishman, 1981). It involves simply asking the interfering person not to interfere, to respect that boundary.

I hypothesized that when a client was having difficulty relating to a part, it might be because of the interference of another part. In those situations, I began asking clients to see whether they could find another part that was influencing them to see the original part in an extreme way. For example, Sally initially called her angry part the Monster and was afraid of it. But when I asked her to find and separate from any parts that were making her feel afraid of it, she found a scared Little Girl. After Sally moved the Little Girl to a safe place in her mind and convinced it to separate its fear from her, she immediately felt sorry for the angry Monster. In addition, the Monster changed; it looked less fierce. After that, the conversation with the angry part was more productive.

The "I" in the Storm

I consistently found that if I asked clients to separate from extreme and polarized parts in this way, most of them could shift quickly into a compassionate or curious state of mind. In that state, they often knew just what to do to help their parts. It seemed that at the core, everyone contained a state of mind that was well suited to leadership. It was through this boundary-making, differentiating process that I encountered what people called their "true Self" or "core Self." This Self felt different to them from their parts. I later discovered that some other approaches described a state of mind like this Self. Generally, however, these approaches saw it as a passive, nonjudgmental observer or witness, in the tradition of Eastern religions, rather than as an active, compassionate leader.

Working with hundreds of clients over more than a decade has led to the conclusion that everyone has a Self, no matter how severe the symptoms or how polarized the internal system. The Self has the clarity of perspective and other qualities needed to lead effectively. When the Self is fully differentiated—for example, through an imagery exercise in which a person is asked to climb a mountain and leave his or her parts in the valley—people universally experience a similar state. They describe feeling "centered," a state of calm well-being and lightheartedness. They feel confident, free, and open-hearted. They describe "being in the present" (i.e., just experiencing with no thinking). They lose their sense of separateness and feel an exhilarating connection to or merger with the universe. This state is similar to what people describe when they meditate.

A similar experience has been reported by participants in a variety of human activities, from various sports to other creative endeavors. Psychologist Mihalyi Csikszentmihalyi (1990) has studied this state of mind, which he calls flow. Flow is characterized by a deep concentration and absence of distracting thoughts; a lack of concern for reward other than the activity itself; a sense of confidence, mastery, and well-being; a loss of the sense of time or of self-consciousness; and a feeling of transcendence. Csikszentmihalyi found that people involved in focused activities around the world described this same state, and he has concluded that it is a universal human experience. Thus it is not just through sitting in meditation that people can experience flow (or what is called Self-leadership in this book). They can be actively engaged in their lives while in this mind set—a state the Buddhists call mindfulness. The Self, then, is not only a passive witness to one's life; it can also be an active leader, both internally and externally.

Particle and Wave

By now, the reader may have noticed that I have described the Self in two different ways: as an active, compassionate inner leader, and as an expansive, boundaryless state of mind. How is it possible for the Self to be both? Some models reconcile this dilemma by differentiating between a "higher Self" and a more mundane, executive Self, or ego. My clinical experience argues against this dichotomy—the Selves of my clients that interact with their parts are the same ones who, when leaving the parts and going up on the mountain, gradually stop thinking and enter a transcendental state. Thus, I believe that the Self is both an individual and a state of consciousness, in the same way that quantum physics has demonstrated that light is both a particle and a wave. That is, photons that make up light sometimes act like particles—like little billiard balls—and other times like waves in a pool of water. They have both qualities (Zohar, 1990). Likewise, the Self can at one time be in its expansive, wavelike state when a person is meditating (fully differentiated from his or her parts) and then shift to being an individual with boundaries (a particle) when that person is trying to help the parts or deal with other people. It is the same Self but in different states.

When in the wave state, a person feels more connection not only to the universe, but also to other people. It is as if, at that level, people's waves can overlap, creating a sense of ultimate commonality and compassion. Thus, helping people differentiate the Self not only helps them harmonize their inner worlds, but also decreases the feeling of difference or isolation among people and builds connectedness.

Self-Protection

How could it be that everyone has this kind of Self? How is it possible that even people who have been severely traumatized or have had virtually no positive parenting in their lives can intuitively know how to be good leaders to their parts? I was confused by these questions until I posed them to some clients who had been severely sexually abused as children. They taught me that a person is organized to protect the Self at all costs. Thus, in the face of trauma or intense emotion, the parts separate the Self from the sensations of their body; they dissociate. If the fear or pain is strong enough, people report feeling as if their Self is taken all the way out of their body to protect it from harm. Consider this description from a rape survivor:

> I left my body at that point. I was over next to the bed, watching this happen. . . . I was standing next to me and there was just this shell on the bed. . . . There was just a feeling of flatness. I was just there. When I repicture the room, I don't picture it from the bed. I picture it from the side of the bed. That's where I was watching from. (Warshaw, 1988, p. 56)

This explains the reports of out-of-body experiences that are so common after trauma. In other survivors' descriptions, the Self, rather than remaining to observe, is moved to a safe limbo-like place where it is oblivious to what is happening. This is why people are frequently amnesic to traumatic or highly intense events. The seat of consciousness—the Self—is elsewhere.

Self-Trust

The problem is that after a person's parts have had to protect the Self in this or in less extreme ways, they lose trust in its ability to lead and increasingly believe that they have to take over. One major goal of therapy becomes helping the client differentiate the Self to the point that the parts can begin to trust it again. For many clients, this happens rapidly and things improve quickly; for others, however, the parts are reluctant to trust the Self and will not separate from it long enough to let it lead. An example of this would be as follows: Suppose that when Sally feared her anger as the Monster and found the Little Girl who was scared of it, that scared child part had refused to separate its feelings from Sally. That is, suppose that her Self had remained undifferentiated from, remained blended with, the Little Girl. Consequently, Sally would have been constrained from knowing and helping the Monster in the way she could have if freed from the Little Girl's fear.

The point here is that whenever the Self is not functioning effectively, it is not because the Self is defective, immature, or inadequate, as some other approaches assume. Instead, the Self has all the necessary qualities for effective leadership,[*] but is constrained by parts that are afraid to differentiate fully from it. This is a difficult assumption for many therapists to accept. Although some therapists who learn this model bring with them a strong intuition about this assumption, others only fully accept it after using the model and seeing it confirmed repeatedly

The Inner Conductor

In addition to the family analogy, I have also used the metaphor of an orchestra to convey the way the parts and Self operate (Beahrs, 1982, also used this metaphor). In this orchestra the individual musicians are analogous to the parts, and the conductor is the Self. I have described this elsewhere as follows:

[*]There are, of course, exceptions to this "fully equipped" assumption. Severe genetic defects or brain injuries can render a person's physiology unable to house this system. Yet the IFS model has been applied effectively to many clients with moderate to severe developmental disabilities. Although they never reach the pinnacle of human potential, they are able to find their parts and relate to them differently.

A good conductor has a sense of the value of each instrument and the ability of every musician, and is so familiar with music theory that he or she can sense precisely the best point in a symphony to draw out one section and mute another. Indeed, it is often as important for a musician to be able to silence his or her instrument at the right time as it is to play the melody skillfully. Each musician, while wanting to spotlight his or her own talent or have the piece played in a way that emphasizes his or her section, has enough respect for the conductor's judgment that he or she remains in the role of following the conductor yet playing as well as possible. This kind of a system is (literally) harmonious.

If, however, the conductor favors the strings and always emphasizes them over the brass, or if the conductor cannot keep the meta-perspective of how the symphony as a whole should sound, or if he or she abdicates and stops conducting altogether, the symphony will become cacophonous. Further, if one of the musicians, lacking the abilities or perspective of a real conductor, tries to take over the conducting, the result would be more incoherence and confusion. (R. C. Schwartz, 1987, p. 31)

Self-Leadership

In sum, a major tenet of IFS is that everyone has at the core, at the seat of consciousness, a Self that is different from the parts. It is the place from which a person observes, experiences, and interacts with the parts and with other people. It contains the compassion, perspective, confidence, and vision required to lead both internal and external life harmoniously and sensitively. It is not just a passive observing state, but can be an actor in both inner and outer dramas. Because most of us have had experiences in which we learned not to trust our Selves, its resources are often obscured by the various extremes of our parts. In addition, while through imagery I can see my parts, I cannot see my Self because it is the me that is doing the seeing, and in that sense it is invisible to me.

For these reasons, people are likely to be identified with their parts and unaware of their Selves. It is easy to have a poor "self-concept" if when one goes inside one sees or feels only these wild and warring denizens. Once clients become aware that their Selves rather than their parts are at their core, and they experience their differentiated Selves, they feel better about life. One major goal of the model, then, is to help each client differentiate the Self as quickly as possible so that it can regain its leadership status. When Self-leadership is available, the parts respond quickly. The client's Self can harmonize the client's inner system, with the therapist in the role of collaborator or cotherapist.

Self-leadership is a noncoercive, collaborative style of leadership. The Self will try to understand parts and people and release them from their extreme roles, rather than trying to force them to change. The Self is similar to the description of a good leader given by Lao Tsu in the *Tao Te Ching* centuries ago: "A leader is best when people barely know that he exists, not so good when they obey and acclaim him, worst when they despise him. Of a good leader, when his work is done, and his aim fulfilled, the People will say, 'We did this ourselves.'"

Patterns of Parts

As discussed earlier, it is useful to think of an internal system as a collection of related people of different ages, like a tribe. Some of these inner-family members are young, sensitive, and vulnerable children; others are older children, adolescents, and adults. In addition to different ages, they have different temperaments, talents, and desires. In a person whose Self is leading this group and the parts are relating harmoniously, the person will not experience each part distinctly and is likely to feel as if his or her mind is unitary. In this respect, the mind is like any other system, from an anthill to a basketball team to a corporation: When it functions well and all the members are in sync, it will seem like one unit. The individual members still exist and, once separated from the group, remain distinct and autonomous. Yet they are so coordinated that they create a kind of unity.

It is in polarized systems, at any level, that the members stand out in bold relief. This is why troubled people report feeling so fragmented—not necessarily because they have more personalities than "normal" people, but because their personalities are fighting with one another rather than working together. Thus, the goal is not to fuse all these smaller personalities into a single big one. It is instead to restore leadership, balance, and harmony, so that each part can take its preferred, valuable role.

Why are parts forced into extreme and destructive roles? How do polarized inner systems evolve? What interferes with Self-leadership? These are the questions that will inform the rest of this chapter.

Why Parts Take On Extreme Roles

Family Imbalances

As any human system evolves, it will be strongly affected by its environment. A family is influenced by mainstream U.S. culture to favor those children who show ambition and independence, while disdaining those who seem easily hurt and dependent. The parent who makes more money will have more esteem and power than the other parent. These cultural biases create imbalances within families: Some members are given more resources, influence, and responsibilities than others of similar age or role. Many of these families are also imbued with patriarchal values, so that males automatically receive more of these qualities than females.

The same process is evident at the intrapsychic level. A client's family will value and embrace some parts of him or her while disdaining others. The client, in turn, is likely to adopt the same attitudes toward these parts, setting up internal imbalances. This is a key IFS principle: People will relate to their parts in much the same way their parents related to those same parts of them.

For example, a female client's parents may stress the importance of pleasing others and looking good, while shaming their daughter when she shows anger. As a result, she allows the parts of her that worry about the approval of others to dominate her life and to exclude parts that want her to assert herself. The approval-seeking parts have too much responsibility, influence, and access to resources, whereas the assertive parts have too little.

Polarization

Imbalanced systems, whether internal or external, will tend to polarize. That is, members of the system will be forced to leave their preferred, valuable roles and take on roles that are either competing with or opposed to those of other members. Parents become enemies, siblings become rivals, parts become antagonists. Each member of the polarization is afraid that if he or she backs down, the other will win or the system will be damaged.

Paul Watzlawick and his colleagues (1974) used a nautical metaphor, which I embellish here, to illustrate polarization in systems. They conjured up an image of "two sailors hanging out of either side of a sailboat in order to steady it: the more the one leans overboard, the more the other has to compensate for the instability created by other's attempts at stabilizing the boat, while the boat itself would be quite steady if not for their acrobatic efforts at steadying it" (p. 36). As I see it, both sailors have left their preferred, valuable roles and are in positions that are destructive to the well-being of the boat, making it susceptible to capsizing. Both are also rigidly limited in their positions. Each has to remain extreme in proportion to the extremes of the other; each can move only in relation to the moves of the other. The irony is that neither likes the role he or she is in and both wish to return to harmony, yet each has valid reasons to fear the consequences of unilaterally leaving his or her position. The boat *would* tip over if either party did move in.

Each sailor is correct in believing that if he or she moves in, the boat will topple because the other will still be leaning out. The only solution is for them both to move in at the same time. Since they do not trust each other, the only way for this to happen is for a third party they both trust to assure each that if one moves in, the other will also. If they had a trusted captain, the captain could coax each to come down off the railing simultaneously. Once released from the strain and constraint of the polarization, each sailor can move about the boat freely and can return to a valuable and enjoyable role, trusting the captain to steer a safe and mutually beneficial course.

To pursue another version of this analogy, let us return to Sally. Many of Sally's parts were polarized in this way. For example, she constantly heard from a voice that pushed her to work, both at her job and in her apartment. If she sat still for any time, this striving part would criticize her for being lazy and remind her of all the things that needed to be done. I had Sally ask the Striver what it was afraid would happen if it did not keep her in constant motion, running her to the point of exhaustion. It said she would get depressed and not get out of bed. Indeed, Sally reported that whenever she paused from this frenetic pace, she became sad, sometimes remaining withdrawn in her apartment for days. "It's like when I slow down, sadness catches up with me."

In its own defense, Sally's Sad One told her that because the Striver was so dominating, the Sad One had to seize any moment of weakness to bring Sally to a grinding halt and hold her down. As soon as it let her get going again, the Striver would reclaim her and would obliterate any sad thoughts or feelings. Thus, each part believed that if it became less extreme, the other would take over—in effect, sinking the boat. These parts were deadlocked. Neither could become less extreme without the assurance that the other would follow suit, and each would resist such a suggestion unless it received that assurance.

Lacking this systemic awareness, many people around Sally, including another therapist, had given her a common-sense prescription: "Why don't you slow down and stop running yourself ragged?" They didn't know that they were inadvertently siding with the Sad One, and consequently making the Striver all the more extreme. Until therapists and others understand the nature of polarization, they will constantly make such mistakes. Just like people in a family or countries in international politics, parts cannot and will not change unilaterally. This points to the importance of viewing a part in the context of the system in which it is embedded. It also demonstrates how a systemic perspective allows parts to change more efficiently and with less coercion than views that do not understand internal politics.

In addition, polarizations tend to be self-confirming, so that even small differences can quickly escalate. The more Sally excluded the part that held her sadness, the more it felt abandoned, hopeless, and sad; the more the Striver believed the Sad One should be exiled, the sadder the Sad One became, and so on. This is the ubiquitous positive feedback loop or vicious circle that is so central to systems thinking. With a systemic awareness, parts can depolarize quickly, as each sees that its assumptions about the other are false.

Parts will not remain depolarized and harmonious for long if the imbalances that contribute to their polarization are not changed as well. Not only did Sally's striving and sad parts need to get to know each other differently and leave their extremes behind; the Striver needed to be given less responsibility, less influence, and fewer resources, and the Sad One needed more. Balance and harmony are intricately linked goals of IFS therapy, and one cannot be achieved without the other.

As is made clear by the boat example, however, achieving harmony and balance in the crew is not possible without effective leadership. Fortunately, everyone already has a capable boat captain in the Self. Once differentiated from her parts, Sally's Self was able to help her Striver and Sad One meet together and end their battle for her soul. Ultimately the Striver shifted into the role of advisor, setting reasonable goals and strategizing their achievement. Once the Sad One got the attention it craved, it no longer felt chronically sad or alone, and brought a child-like zest and joy to Sally's life.

To summarize, the values and interaction patterns within a person's family of origin will shape his or her internal relations. The person will give some parts more and other parts less resources, influence, and responsibility. These imbalances will trigger polarizations that can quickly escalate and chronically stress or paralyze a person's internal system. By achieving Self-leadership, however, a person can quickly depolarize internal relationships, releasing the parts to find and adopt their preferred, valuable roles.

Trauma

Imbalanced family values and interactions are not the only forces that create polarizations, however. When people are rejected, abandoned, shocked, scared, or abused (physically, sexually, or emotionally), their inner systems can easily polarize also. My colleagues and I have been taught by hundreds of traumatized clients the common patterns of inner imbalance and polarization that such intense episodes can bring.

When any human system—a family, company, or country—suffers some kind of threatening or overwhelming trauma, the system organizes to protect its leadership as well as its most sensitive and vulnerable members. Internal families operate in this same way. Let us return to the analogy of a tribe of inner people of various ages and degrees of vulnerability, led by a Self. In the face of danger, the tribe moves the Self to a place of safety, and certain parts come forward to deal with the danger.

It may be useful to compare a person's Self and parts to the functioning of a country. As another country threatens to attack, the president is moved to a special place of safety (in the United States, he or she is in a jet flying above the fray), civilians are sent to shelters, and the military takes over. If through the crisis the president stays calm, and provides the strength and comfort that leads to a satisfactory resolution of the crisis, then the trauma may increase the people's trust in their leader. If, however, the president cannot prevent the devastation of the country, the president loses credibility, and military leaders are likely to remain in power to protect and manage the country.

Internal families organize in a similar way. As mentioned above, physically or emotionally traumatized clients have taught us that before or during a trauma, for protective reasons, the Self is separated from the sensations of a person's body to varying degrees, depending on the perceived severity of the trauma. Some of the older, less vulnerable inner-tribe members take control and try to protect the system. They do this in a variety of ways. Some may want the person to lash out; others try to execute an escape; still others try to make the person freeze and become totally passive. All of these protectors try to numb the person, to minimize the sensations reaching the Self and other parts.

Despite these efforts, the youngest, most sensitive, and most vulnerable members of the inner tribe can be powerfully affected by the traumatic experience. They feel most acutely the emotions and sensations (pain, terror, despair, abandonment, betrayal, etc.). They can be so stimulated by the experience that it is as if their circuits overload and they become frozen in time at the point of the trauma. When this is the case, these parts live thereafter as if they are still fixed in that situation, with all its feelings and sensations. By contrast, if the Self is able to help avert extreme damage during or after the trauma, and is able to comfort these hurt parts and help them out of their frozen state, then trust in the Self's leadership may increase and the system will not necessarily polarize. In such cases, the trauma builds rather than destroys character.

What determines whether or not the Self is able to lead the tribe through the trauma? If the victim is a child, much depends on the reactions of those around him or her. For example, in the aftermath of the event, if the child is returned to safety, is helped to accept and understand what happened, and is given love and comfort, then his or her Self is able to respond in the same way to hurt parts—with love, comfort, and acceptance. In this best-case scenario, the hurt parts will heal in the sense that they will know the person appreciates what they went through and still values them. They will not remain stuck at the moment of the event; instead, they will be released from the pain and memories, and will take their preferred, valuable roles in the internal system.

On the other hand, in a case where the Self is impotent to protect the system and not allowed to help those most traumatized afterward, parts lose trust in the Self's leadership and become overprotective of the Self and of the parts who were hurt. Such people become dominated by their protectors and often report feeling no sense of Self. They are often seen by therapists as having little or no ego strength. It is sometimes difficult but always important with such a client to remember that the Self is still there, although it is not allowed to use its resources, which are obscured by protective parts and separated from the person's body.

It is like a solar eclipse. In ancient times, when the moon moved in front of the sun, people used to fear the darkness and believe the sun was gone forever. Traumatized people often believe that their sun is gone. Many feel disconnected from life, psychically homeless, as if their spirits were missing or had died and they were just going through the motions of living. The IFS model can help such a person see that the Self is still there and can shine again.

The Three-Group System: Exiles, Managers, and Firefighters

The processes described above organize human systems into three groups. One group tends to be highly protective, strategic, and interested in controlling the environment to keep things safe. In an internal family, the members of this group are called the "managers." Another group contains the most sensitive members of the system. When injured or outraged, the members of this group will be imprisoned by the managers for their own and the larger system's protection; they become the "exiles." A third group reacts powerfully and automatically when the exiles are upset, to try to stifle or soothe those feelings. Its members are called the "firefighters." In many internal systems, polarizations exist among these three groups and also within them.

The way many people react to trauma sets up a polarization between parts that are exiled and those that are trying to protect and run the system. The more the hurt, rageful, or sexually charged exiles are shut out, the more extreme they become, and the more the managers and firefighters legitimately fear their release. So they resort to more extreme methods of suppression. The more the exiles are suppressed, the more they try to break out, and all three groups become victims of an escalating vicious circle. Judith Herman (1992) describes such cycles:

[A trauma survivor] finds herself caught between the extremes of amnesia or of reliving the trauma, between floods of intense, overwhelming feelings and arid states of no feeling at all, between irritable, impulsive action and complete inhibition of action. The instability produced by these periodic alternations further exacerbates the traumatized person's sense of unpredictability and helplessness. (p. 47)

Exiles

Commonly, children are taught to fear and hide their pain or terror. The adults react to a hurt child's feelings in the same extreme way they react to their own hurt inner-child parts—with impatience, denial, criticism, revulsion or distraction. Managerial parts of the child soon learn to adopt these attitudes and constrain the Self from taking care of the younger tribe members. This makes many people quite vulnerable to polarization from trauma. They become inclined to try to forget about painful events as soon as possible, which means pushing their hurting parts out of awareness. In this way, insult is added to the injury of these child parts. They are like children who are hurt and then are rejected and abandoned because they are hurt. They become the exiles, closeted away and enshrouded with burdens of unlovability, shame, or guilt.

Like any oppressed group, these exiles become increasingly extreme and desperate, looking for opportunities to break out of their prison and tell their stories. In this effort they give the person flashbacks or nightmares or sudden, fleeting tastes of pain or fear. Like abandoned children, many of the exiles desperately want to be cared for and loved. They constantly look for someone who might rescue and redeem them.

Moreover, the exiles can become receptacles for feelings that other parts do not want to carry. That is, the parts that have to run the person's life (the managers) transfer to these exiles their burdens of fear, pain, shame, or other emotions that interfere with managerial functioning. Consequently, the exiles want to rid themselves of these excess emotions and will try to give them to other parts or to the Self at any opportunity.

In this state of distress and neediness, exiles may endanger the person. While they are frozen in the past and locked away behind inner walls, they are less vulnerable to being hurt by events in the present. Bringing them out not only floods the person with unpleasant memories and feelings, but also makes him or her more fragile and easily injured. In addition, when these exiles take control they often lead the person into danger. They seek a redeemer who resembles the person who rejected them initially (or even the actual abuser), in order to find the love and protection they believe will heal the pain of rejection and finally make them feel safe. Often these parts will pay virtually any price for even small amounts of love, acceptance, or protection, or for the hope of redemption. In return, they are willing to endure (and, indeed, often believe they deserve) more degradation and abuse. Many such clients repeatedly enter and have difficulty exiting, abusive relationships. Their exiles keep taking over and exposing them to being hurt again and again.

Thus, managers have good reasons to fear exiles, who are hurt and vulnerable. Frequently other parts are also perceived as dangerous and are forced into exile. These often include parts that are enraged about the trauma, particularly when it involved abuse, and want revenge. In addition, when the abuse involved sex, the parts that were sexually stimulated during it are seen as disgusting or extremely dangerous and are locked in the inner prison. They are associated with the abuser, and their existence makes the person believe that, deep down, he or she is as bad as the abuser.

Managers

Thus, managers live in fear of the escape of exiles. They try to avoid any interactions or situations that might activate an exile's attempts to break out or leak feelings, sensations, or memories into consciousness. Different managers adopt different strategies. It must be kept in mind that managers are forced into roles they do not enjoy but believe are necessary. I describe some of the common managerial roles here.

Often there is a manager that tries to keep the person in control of all relationships or situations, afraid that the smallest slight or frightening surprise might activate one of the young hurt parts. This manager may be highly intellectual and effective at solving problems, but is also obsessed with pushing away all feeling. Clients often call this part the Controller, or something similar. Relatedly, this or another part may strive for career success or wealth, so as to put the person in a position of power and to distract him or her from feelings. To motivate the person, the Striver is often a bitingly critical taskmaster, never satisfied with performance or outcome.

Another managerial part often becomes perfectionistic about the person's appearance and behavior, believing that if the person is perfect and pleases everyone, he or she will not be abandoned or hurt. With bulimic clients, this Evaluator focuses on weight, constantly calling them fat or gluttonous. Another manager may try to keep the person in a victim's role to ensure that other people will take care of him or her. This manager, the Dependent One, keeps the person appearing helpless, injured, and passive.

Another manager tries to avoid interpersonal risk, particularly situations that could arouse anger, sexuality, or fear. This Passive Pessimist can make the person totally apathetic and withdrawn, so that he or she does not try to get close to anyone. This part often erodes the person's self-confidence and sabotages performance, so that he or she will not have the courage to pursue goals. Or the part may look for and accentuate any flaws in an object of desire, in order to undermine attempts to obtain it. In people who have been severely abused, this part can become an inner Terrorist, taking on qualities of the abuser and scaring the exiles into making the person even more withdrawn.

Many women are socialized to rely heavily on a manager called the Caretaker, who, when extreme, makes them always sacrifice their own needs so as to focus on and care for others. This part is likely to criticize a woman for being selfish if she ever asserts herself. Other common managerial roles include the hyperaroused Worrier or Sentry, who feels in constant jeopardy, is on continuous alert for danger, and flashes worst-case scenarios in front of a person as he or she contemplates risk; the Denier, who distorts perceptions to keep the person from seeing and responding to risky feedback; and the Entitled One, who encourages the person to get whatever he or she wants, no matter who is wronged by the action (men are often socialized to rely on this manager).

Caretaker

Worrier

Denier

Entitled One

The point to remember is that the primary purpose of all managers is to keep the exiles exiled, both for the protection of the exiles themselves and the protection of the system from them. That is, the goal is to keep the feared feelings and thoughts from spilling over the inner walls, so that the system remains safe and the person is able to function in life. The managers' main strategy is to pre-empt the activation of exiles by keeping the person in control or out of danger (unknown or unpredictable situations) at all times and pleasing those on whom the person depends.

In order to maintain this kind of internal and external control, some managers can give the person the outward appearance and substance of success, providing the drive and focus to gain impressive academic, career, or monetary achievements. Success not only brings control over relationships and choices, but also can serve to distract from or compensate for the person's inner shame, fear, sadness, or despair. On the other hand, if the client is dominated by a Passive Pessimist, Dependent One, or Worrier, his or her life may be characterized by a series of half-hearted attempts and failures, which provide protection from responsibility or disappointment. Other common managerial tools or manifestations include: obsessions, compulsions, reclusiveness, passivity, emotional detachment and sense of unreality, phobias, panic attacks, somatic complaints, depressive episodes, hyperalertness, and nightmares.

The rigidity and severity of these various managerial strategies will match the degree to which the managers think (correctly or not) that the person is in danger of being reinjured. Contributing to their rigidity and extremeness is the fact that they have more responsibility than they are equipped to handle. They not only have to deal with what they perceive as a dangerous outside world; they also have their finger in the dike that contains the exiles, and are desperate to protect the Self from these internal and external threats. In this position, managers are neglected, suffering, and scared, like parentified children in a dysfunctional family.

This passage from Alice Miller's (1981) *The Drama of the Gifted Child* illustrates a parental child's predicament, which is identical to the predicament of many manager parts in internal families. Miller's patient was the eldest child of a professional woman:

> I was the jewel in my mother's crown. She often said: "Maja can be relied upon, she will cope." And I did cope. I brought up the smaller children for her so that she could get on with her professional career. She became more famous, but I never saw her happy. How often I longed for her in the evenings. The little ones cried and I comforted them but I myself never cried. Who would have wanted a crying child? I could only win my mother's love if I was competent, understanding, and controlled, if I never questioned her actions nor showed her how much I missed her. (p. 68)

When one gets to know the striving, perfectionistic, and approval-seeking managers inside a client, those parts often describe similar feelings of having to hide their own loneliness and misery, because someone has to keep the person's life under control. Like the exiles, they also want to be nurtured and healed, but they believe they have to hide those vulnerabilities and sacrifice themselves for the system. The more competent they become, the more the system relies on them, and the more they become overwhelmed with their responsibilities and power. They come to believe that they alone are responsible for any success and safety the person has experienced, and increasingly lose trust in the leadership of the Self.

Firefighters

There will be times when, despite the best efforts of the managers, the exiles are activated and threaten to break out and take over. When this happens, another group of parts leaps into action to try to contain or extinguish the feelings, sensations, or images. I call this group the "firefighters" because they react automatically whenever an exiled part is activated. It is as if an alarm goes off and they frantically mobilize to put out the fire of feelings. They do whatever they believe necessary to help the person dissociate from or douse dreaded, exiled feelings, with little regard for the consequences of their methods.

The techniques of firefighters often include numbing activities such as self-mutilation, binge eating, drug or alcohol abuse, excessive masturbation, or promiscuity. When activated, a firefighter will try to take control of the person so thoroughly that he or she feels nothing but an urgent compulsion to engage in a dissociative or self-soothing activity. These firefighters can make the person self-absorbed and demanding (narcissistic), driven insatiably to grab more material things for himself or herself than anyone else. Firefighter activities also sometimes include the numbing and protectiveness of rage, the exhilaration and indulgence of stealing, or the comfort of suicidal thoughts or attempts.

Although firefighters have the same basic goal as managers—to keep the exiles exiled—their roles and strategies are quite different from, and often in conflict with, those of managers. Managers strive to prevent the activation of exiles by keeping the person in control at all times and by pleasing everyone, particularly those on whom the person depends. They are often highly rational and planful, able to anticipate and pre-empt activating situations. Firefighters, on the other hand, usually react after the activation of exiles has occurred. They take the person out of control and displease everyone around him or her. They are often impulsive, unthinking, and reactive. Whereas managers tend to react to activated exiles by trying to shut them out more, firefighters are more likely to find something that will calm or appease the exiles—to douse the fire.

Managers and firefighters, then, are strange and uncomfortable bedfellows. Managers rely on firefighters and call on them when necessary, but afterward scornfully attack them for having made the person indulgent, weak-willed, endangered, and insensitive to others. Firefighters, then, often bring a barrage of criticism from inner managers, as well as from the managers in the external people around the client. This disapproval will reactivate the exiles, which in turn triggers the firefighters again, and so on. Thus, the person is caught in another escalating vicious cycle: The more the exiles try to break through, the more the managers and firefighters desperately try to contain them, but their containment attempts themselves activate the exiles.

Most people, even those who never were severely hurt, are organized internally according to these three groups: managers, firefighters, and exiles. This is because most people are socialized to exile various parts of themselves, and once that process begins, the managerial and firefighter roles become necessary. The kind of symptoms a client experiences will be related to which of these groups dominates them. For example, people with various addictions are often dominated by firefighters; those who are chronically depressed are often dominated by managers; and those who experience bouts of intense sadness or fear may be dominated frequently by exiles. The length of treatment and the difficulty of change are related to how much trust exists within the system for a person's Self and how polarized the parts are, rather than to the severity of symptoms themselves. Generally, the worse and the longer someone was hurt, the more polarized the person's system is, and the less trust exists for Self-leadership.

Burdens

Thus far, I have discussed how parts are forced into extreme roles because they are polarized with other parts, because they are protecting other parts, or because they are frozen in time. There is one other reason that bears discussion. Parts often take on extreme ideas, behaviors, or feelings derived from extreme events or interactions with others in a person's life, and carry these like transferred burdens that organize and constrain them.

Parts are particularly susceptible to absorbing these transferred burdens when the person is young. A young child cannot survive unaided, and consequently is highly dependent on his or her parents. The child believes, often correctly, that the penalty for the parents' not valuing or caring about him or her is abandonment, severe harm, or death. As a result, children are very sensitive to messages from parents regarding their evaluation of them. When those messages are consistently reassuring, this hypersensitivity abates quickly, and a child's internal system is not constrained by this issue from developing harmoniously. If, however, the family in which a child develops is imbalanced and polarized, the child is likely to receive inconsistent messages, at best, regarding worth during this period of high dependence.

Worthlessness and the Need for Redemption

When a child is uncertain or pessimistic about his or her value, the child strives to understand and become what is perceived as pleasing to the parents. The normal need for approval becomes a craving and children take to heart extreme messages they are given about their worth. If a child is told, verbally or nonverbally, that he or she is of little value, young parts of the child organize their beliefs around that premise. They become desperate for redemption in the eyes of the person who gave these messages. Thereafter these parts carry the burden of worthlessness, which makes them believe that no one can love them—a belief they will maintain no matter what feedback is received from others. It is as if the person who devalued the child stole his or her self-esteem and holds title to it. The child then believes that to survive, he or she must get it back from the person who took it away. In this way, the person on whom the child depends becomes the redeemer. And this is not always a child's parent, but can be anyone on whom he or she depends.

These burdened young parts exert a powerful influence over the person's intimate relationships as they constantly seek redemption—the lifting of what feels like a curse of unlovability. They will return to the person who stole their self-esteem in this quest, or they will find someone who resembles that person. Often this results in a history of abusive or unsatisfying relationships.

Other Burdens

In this same scenario, other of the child's parts are likely to take on qualities of the person who stole his or her self-esteem and sense of safety. These parts are so desperate to win the approval of that person that they mimic him or her in an effort to make the child become more acceptable. These generally become managerial parts within the child; they are often inner critics or moralizers who carry the burden of perfectionism, believing that if they can make the child perfect, he or she will finally be redeemed.

In similar ways, parts take on other burdens. Commonly transferred burdens include having to protect another family member; having to be a great success; and believing that one will never succeed or that the world is very dangerous. Virtually any extreme part of a parent or other authority can be mimicked by these approval-craving parts of a child. It is not uncommon to see the same burden being passed from generation to generation in families—a process to be discussed in Chapter 6.

This burden-transferring process is the aspect of the IFS model that is the most similar to what has been called "introjection." One important difference is that it is only the burden that is introjected, not the essence of the part. That is, once the burden has been lifted, the part will be released from its influence and will be better able to pursue its preferred, constructive role. If instead the part is viewed as merely a mental introject, its valuable qualities and its ability to change will be underestimated.

Sally Revisited

To make this discussion more concrete, let us return once again to Sally. As mentioned earlier, Sally alternated between long periods of driven activity and brief episodes of intense sadness and loneliness. This pattern reflected the domination of striving managers, broken periodically by exiled, hurt child parts. She also was building a history of troubled relationships with men, and found that the frequency and intensity of her bulimic episodes corresponded to these patterns. That is, when she was not involved with a man and obsessed with work, her bingeing followed a regular schedule (usually once per day when she got home from work) that interfered very little with her activities. During this period, the binges were used by her Striver as a palliative, to quiet the exiles' loneliness so that they would not interfere with her activity.

Once Sally gave in to the exiles' pressure and began dating, the inner tension mounted, and her bulimic episodes increased and became less predictable. Now the bulimia was used by her Passive Pessimist to prove to her that she was sick, defective, and disgusting, and had no business getting close to men. The closer she got, the more symptomatic she became until she began withdrawing emotionally from the relationship, leaving the man feeling confused and angry. His anger become more evidence that she should escape, and ultimately she would stop answering his calls until he gave up.

Despite the fact that she was the initiator of these breakups, they always left Sally feeling raw and desperately sad. Her exiles, feeling deprived and rejected once again, would sometimes break out again for weeks. Convinced by her Pessimist that they would never get the love they craved, her exiles kept her at home except to go to the grocery store, but held her in intense misery and emptiness. These were times when she binged and purged wildly, violently, as her firefighters scrambled to douse the roaring blaze of emotion that had spread out of control. Eventually the fires burned themselves out and her managers regained control, helped her find a new job (since she lost several as a result of these withdrawals), and refocused her on work, until she met another man and the sequence would repeat itself.

Within this long sequence were embedded several similar, shorter sequences. For example, Sally had frequent contact with her parents, who, as the reader will recall, were trying to improve their marriage in an effort to let Sally grow up. Despite her relief at no longer having to protect her parents, many of these visits left Sally confused and upset, even though they were full of pleasant interactions. Her exiles missed the special closeness with her father and were jealous to see that he was now clearly more connected to her mother. No matter how hard Sally berated herself for having what she considered disgusting and irrational reactions, she could not shake a sense of betrayal and displacement at no longer being the apple of Daddy's eye.

Sally's reaction to this craving for her father's approval illustrates how managers also polarize with one another regarding how best to deal with the exiles. Sally's Striver insisted that her father no longer cared about her, so she should move on by building a career. It also said that her parents caused her bulimia and that the healthiest thing to do was to get away from them. On the other hand, her Passive Pessimist, out of worry that she would fail in the world, lobbied for the opposite course. It tried to use the bulimia as proof that she could not make it on her own and had to move back home.

What I hope is clear from this example is that, although firefighters were always involved in creating Sally's binges, they were triggered by other parts for a variety of reasons. The bulimia might be used to soothe and dissociate, but also to make a case for her inadequacy, in order to prevent rejection or to motivate her to leave home. For this reason, simple, single explanations of why Sally binged and purged are inadequate. Different parts used her symptoms for different purposes, and for her to discard her symptoms, she needed to release each of these and other constraints.

How did Sally's system develop these polarizations? As I worked with her parts, they provided some of the answers, which also were not simple. At one level, Sally's internal family reflected the imbalances and polarizations of her external family. Her father was the embodiment of a Striver, who pushed himself and those around him to excel and look perfect. He bristled when his wife or daughter complained about anything, and he strongly believed in the power of positive thinking. He wanted to believe that Sally was perpetually happy, so she tried to wear a smile around him and to keep her sadness hidden. He was also an impatient, driven man who interacted with Sally mainly in regard to her performance at school, and never seemed satisfied even though she did well.

Sally's mother seemed chronically bitter and was less successful than Sally at wearing a happy mask around the father. She frequently complained about his long hours at work, both to him and to Sally. She also was very concerned about Sally's appearance, criticizing her clothes and her hair style. During preadolescence, Sally gained weight to the point of plumpness, and her mother began nagging her to eat less. Sally went on a crash diet during her junior year in high school, and after struggling down to a trim 105 pounds, she began to purge out of fear of gaining.

When Sally and her mother were not fighting over her eating or other picky issues, they were constant companions. Sally cheered up her mother in various ways and buried her own despair. This lasted until her junior year in high school, when Sally began to withdraw for long periods into her room, where she was secretly bingeing and purging.

From these family influences, Sally's parts inherited the burden of her father's striving perfectionism, her mother's critical evaluation of her appearance, and the disdain that both her parents demonstrated for her assertive and sad parts. Parts of her also felt responsible for each parent's happiness, and (particularly in her mother's case) always believed that she was failing in that role. These burdens set up the roles for many of the managerial parts that ran her life until her junior year, when her Passive Pessimist took over, along with the firefighter that made her binge to protect her from all this pressure. Thus, Sally's managers were divided between those that wanted her to please others and be successful, and those that tried to hide her behind the walls of her room and her bulimia.

Because of these family attitudes, Sally would have had to exile her angry and sensitive, lonely parts even if she had never suffered any severe traumas. The traumas she did suffer only made their exile more oppressive. When in therapy some of her hurt child parts showed where they were frozen in the past, one of them showed a time when, at age 5, Sally's mother was hospitalized for what Sally later learned was a "nervous breakdown." Sally was terrified to find her mother suddenly gone, and no one explained to her what was happening. Her father seemed preoccupied and uncomfortable in her presence. Her grandmother stayed with her but was not a nurturing woman. When her mother returned, she acted as if nothing was wrong and she had just been on a short trip. This Little Girl part was frozen in that time of confusion, loneliness, and fear of having been abandoned. She thought she had done something to make her mother leave, and so was also fraught with guilt.

Another exile showed Sally a scene in which, at age 7, a teenage cousin made her touch his penis. This was an event that Sally had no memory of until the exile took her back to it. This 7-year-old lived there amid all the disgust, shame, and confusion. She desperately wanted to be rescued by her parents and felt powerless and dirtied; she was too ashamed and afraid to tell anyone.

There were several other traumatic stuck places, each holding an exile in its grip. During each of these past episodes, Sally's managers had left the part that suffered the most in that place and time, and tried to move the rest of the system forward by forgetting about the abandoned part. As each exile was retrieved from its frozen place (in a process to be described in later chapters), her managers and firefighters were gradually able to let go of their burdens and extreme roles, and find more valuable and enjoyable roles.

Sally's internal family reflected the imbalances and polarizations of her external family; it was also influenced by traumatic episodes, which left parts frozen in the past and burdened with extreme feelings and beliefs. As a result, Sally's inner and outer worlds were tension filled. Her system's solution was either to binge, purge, and withdraw, or to work compulsively. Amid comparable environments, other people's internal families find other solutions, which run the gamut of syndromes described in diagnostic manuals. After working with a wide range of problems, one can see the same three-group system of parts involved in each. The differences in presentation are determined by differences in firefighter activity, managerial strategy, or exile craving.

Summary

This chapter has presented a large number of principles. To help organize them, I outline some key assumptions of the IFS model.

Multiplicity

It is the nature of the human mind to be subdivided into an indeterminate number of subpersonalities called parts (most clients identify and work with between 5 and 15 parts through the course of therapy). These parts are conceptualized as inner people of different ages, temperaments, talents, and desires, who together form an internal family or tribe. This internal family organizes itself in the same way as other human systems and reflects the organization of the systems around it.

Parts exist from birth, either in potential or in actuality. That is, multiplicity is inherent in the nature of the mind, rather than being the result of the introjection of external phenomena (although parts may for various reasons take on or get stuck with images or behaviors of significant people), or the result of fragmentation through trauma of the once-unitary personality (although trauma will polarize the already existing parts).

All parts are valuable and want to play constructive inner roles. They are forced into extreme and destructive roles by external influences and by the self-perpetuating nature of inner polarizations and imbalances. They will gratefully find or return to preferred, valuable roles once they believe it is safe to do so.

The Self

In addition to this collection of parts, at the core of everyone is a Self, which is the seat of consciousness. From birth this Self has all the necessary qualities of good leadership, such as compassion, perspective, curiosity, acceptance, and confidence. As a result, the Self makes the best internal leader, and will engender inner balance and harmony if it is allowed by the parts to lead. A person's parts are organized to protect the Self at all costs and will remove it from danger and from leadership in the face of trauma. Parts will then blend their extreme feelings or thoughts with the Self, obscuring its leadership qualities, and causing it to be separated from the sensations of the person's body.

The Self comes fully equipped to lead and does not have to develop through stages or be borrowed from or strengthened by the therapist. It is also not merely a passive observer or witness state; instead, once differentiated from the parts, it becomes an active, compassionate, and collaborative leader. When the Self is differentiated from the parts (i.e., has separated from their feelings and thoughts), regains their trust, and returns to the body, then Self-leadership is restored.

Self-Leadership

All systems—families, companies, nations—function best when leadership is clearly designated, respected, fair, and capable. Internal families are no different. When the Self is unconstrained, it will lead in the sense of caring for and depolarizing the parts in an equitable and compassionate way; leading discussions with the parts regarding major decisions in selecting the direction of the person's life; and dealing with the external world.

When Self-leadership is achieved, the parts do not disappear (although their extreme roles do, as does the rigid three-group system). Instead, they remain to advise, remind, work on solutions to problems, lend talents or emotions, or otherwise help; each has a different, valuable role and set of abilities. Generally they cooperate rather than compete or conflict with each other, and when conflicts arise, the Self mediates. When this is the case, the person is less aware of the existence of the parts, because the system operates harmoniously and (as in any harmonious system) each individual member is less noticeable. That is, the person will feel more unified, with a sense of continuity and integration.

This is not to suggest that the goal is to never have a part take over leadership temporarily. In many situations, certain parts have abilities that make them the best leaders. At other times it is fun or thrilling to let some parts take over. The point is that when Self-leadership is restored parts can still take over, but not for the same protective or polarized reasons, and with the permission of the Self. They will also withdraw from leadership when the Self requests it.

Polarization

Many past or current events can affect the leadership, balance, and harmony of a person's internal system. The most common of such influences include family-of-origin attitudes and interactions, and traumatic experiences. When because of these influences parts take over leadership from the Self, take on burdens, become frozen in the past, or are otherwise forced into extreme roles, the internal relations shift from harmony and polarize. As one part shifts to an extreme role and unbalances the distribution of resources, influence, and responsibilities, another will take an opposing or competing role. Because they tend to be self-confirming, these polarizations are likely to escalate in the absence of effective leadership. That is, the negative assumptions each part has about the other are continually confirmed, as each part becomes more extreme to try to counter or defeat the other. Polarizations lead to coalitions in which groups of parts unite in opposition or competition with other groups.

The Three-Group Ecology

Thus, highly polarized internal systems are rigid and delicate ecologies that will react severely to being disrupted. Trying to change any one part without considering the network in which it is embedded is likely to activate what has been called "resistance," but is actually a natural and often necessary ecological reaction. For this reason, it is important to have a useful map of these relationships and to be respectful of the valid reasons for which they are so protected.

Restoring Balance, Harmony, and Leadership

Even highly polarized internal systems can heal themselves if the therapist can create a safe, caring environment and can point the person in certain directions. The system already has all the necessary resources, and needs only to release and reorganize those resources. In addition, all parts of the system want to relate harmoniously and will eagerly leave their extreme roles, once convinced it is safe to do so.

If, however, the person lives in a dangerous or otherwise activating environment, this internal harmonizing process will be more difficult and prolonged. Parts will be reluctant to leave their roles if they are constantly activated by interactions with other people. And as the person changes, others may have protective counterreactions to those shifts. For this reason, the therapist and client will be well advised to find and release constraints in the client's external world as well. Chapters 6, 7, and 8 focus on external constraints.

Internal and External Parallels

With the IFS model, then, the client's internal and external worlds comprise one large system, operating according to the same principles and responsive to the same techniques. In addition, because systems that interface come to reflect one another, changes at one level can produce parallel changes at other levels. For example, Sally's internal family reflected the values and structure of her external family. As her external family structure changed (e.g., her parents fought less and became better leaders), this shift had a parallel effect on her internal system. Her managers became less polarized and allowed more Self-leadership. Correspondingly, as Sally's Self kept her parts that worried so much about her parents out of the lead, thereby setting better internal boundaries, her family's boundaries also became clearer and less diffuse.

This recursiveness between and among systems at the internal and external levels has several implications. First, a therapist should not work with a client's internal system without thoroughly considering and addressing the person's external context. Second, a therapist can, for example, work only with a client's external family to improve its leadership without directly addressing the client's internal family, but can still create major internal shifts in leadership (see Chapter 7). Thus, in deciding at what level to focus therapy, one assesses both the external and internal system levels, focuses on whichever level change may be most impactful or expedient, and shifts levels fluidly as indicated. All of this is possible because it seems that human systems at all levels operate according to these same principles of balance, harmony, and leadership.

CHAPTER 3

Case Example

Methods for using the IFS model with individuals are described in Chapters 4 and 5. Those methods will be more understandable if the reader first has a general picture of how this therapy works. This chapter brings to life the concepts of IFS by presenting the course of therapy with an individual. It also offers commentary designed to spotlight common predicaments and patterns.

When she came to me for therapy, Nina was an attractive 27-year-old widow. Her husband had died 2 years earlier, after 3 years of marriage, and she had been reclusive since his death. In our first session, she shamefully confessed to regular ferocious bouts of bingeing and vomiting. They had begun after the funeral and had increasingly dominated her life.

Nina lived alone, and although she felt lonely, she was afraid to be around people until she felt less sad. She did not want to burden friends with her sorrow at the loss of her husband; also since the sorrow was ever-present, she was not up to making small talk. She said she hated the fact that after 2 years, she was still so obsessed with her loss and had not moved on in her life. Increasingly she was thinking that life would never be good again, and consequently that she should commit suicide. The bulimia accentuated her sense of desperation, shame, and hopelessness, and she felt totally at its mercy.

History

Nina was estranged from her own family. Her first-generation Hungarian parents believed that their children should remain obedient and close to the family. She was 10 years younger than her next sibling, and so she witnessed the consequences to her older brother and sister of following those rules. Both of them lived at home until they married at ages 31 and

28, and then they moved into houses one and three doors away from their parents, respectively. Nina watched her sister run to her mother every time she had a fight with her husband. She watched her brother try to become the lawyer her father wanted him to be and wind up a depressed store clerk, dependent financially and emotionally on his parents.

To avoid her siblings' fate, Nina resolved to live and think independently. She was the rebellious one, fighting constantly with her parents (particularly her mother) over dating and curfew. Her father was a hard-working carpenter who left most of the parenting to his wife. He related to the children as the paternal advice giver, and tended to give long, moralistic lectures. He encouraged Nina to pursue her talents in science and go to college—but, of course, to the nearby commuter school, so that she could continue to live at home. Nina's mother thought that more school for her daughter was a waste of time, since Nina should, like her, take care of a family. Nina did attend the commuter college while living with her parents, and continued to fight frequently with her mother.

As long as Nina could remember, her parents had battled with each other. After such fights, her mother complained to any of the children who would listen that they were the only reason she did not leave him. Nina's sister was her mother's primary confidante in these matters; Nina tried to avoid involvement in them, but sometimes found herself defending her father's actions.

Early into her dating experience in college, Nina fell in love with Tom. He was 7 years older than Nina and Greek—two qualities that ensured disapproval from her parents. He was the first person who really seemed to care about her, however. With his encouragement, after graduating from college Nina took a full-time job and moved into her own apartment, sneaking her belongings out one weekend while her parents were out of town. Their reaction was worse than she had dreamed it would be. Her father took it as a personal affront: If a girl left her parents' home before marriage, it meant that she could not stand them or they could not afford to keep her. He felt deserted and refused to speak to her. Her sister by this time had divorced her husband, and in contrast to Nina (but like her mother) was quite overweight. Her sister seized the opportunity to shift out of the failure position, becoming the most vocal in her outrage over what Nina was "doing to her parents" by moving out. Nina became the family outcast; she was aware that her mother and sister spent hours criticizing her.

After a year of independent living, Nina married Tom. Tom's widowed mother became a surrogate parent to her. Nina came to depend on Tom and his mother for everything—a situation that Tom encouraged. He liked having her lean on him. Nine months into their marriage, however, Tom discovered that he had cancer. For the 2 years before his death, Nina devoted virtually all of her energy to comforting him and helping him fight for his life. She felt terrified and despondent at the prospect of life without Tom, but believed she could not let him or his mother see her that way. She was also shocked and hurt to find that her parents and siblings maintained their distance from her throughout the crisis, although she never directly asked for any help from them. After Tom's death she resented him for encouraging her to depend on him so much and then deserting her, but felt terribly guilty and selfish for entertaining such thoughts.

Context at Beginning of Therapy

Nina tried to fill all of her time with her job as a personal trainer in a health center and with a rigorous exercise regimen. It seemed that whenever she paused even briefly, her depression caught up with her. Her mother-in-law was still constantly mourning the loss of her son with tears and reminiscences, and Nina felt it her duty to continue to console her during her once- or twice-weekly visits to the older woman. The only request Nina denied was to accompany Tom's mother on visits to her son's grave; she was afraid that she could not maintain her facade of strength in that context. Thus, she was in the position of desperately trying to run away from thoughts of her loss, while constantly confronted with it by her mother-in-law. Around her mother-in-law, she pretended to be strong and stoic while feeling overwhelming despair.

As I listened to Nina tell this story, I began asking about the parts of her that were activated by these relationships with her own family and with her mother-in-law. I asked about her vision of what she would like her inner and outer lives to be. I also asked about how constraining these internal and external relationships were. Nina believed that her fear of burdening her mother-in-law was the biggest external constraint, but she attributed the constraining effect of that relationship more to her own parts than to anything the mother-in-law was doing. I decided to respect her request not to involve her mother-in-law in the therapy at that point and to work with Nina individually; we agreed that we might invite others in as needed later.

I felt confident in this decision, partly because it seemed that Nina's context at this time contained enough room for her to change without upsetting any highly reactive people on whom she depended. Unlike many younger or more dependent clients, Nina was not embedded in a family context that constantly activated her parts, or that would be disturbed if she were to get stronger. She was not financially dependent on anyone. She lived alone, rarely saw her family of origin, and was no longer a part of protective sequences with her parents or siblings. Although her visits to her mother-in-law often left her upset, they could be spaced to coordinate with our work. She was not involved in power struggles or any other symptom-maintaining sequences with anyone (except for herself) in regard to her bulimia; indeed, she believed that no one else knew of her secret. She felt most constrained by her internal system, so we began at that level.

Over the 14 sessions I had with Nina (10 weekly, shifting to 4 at 2-week intervals), the spotlight of therapy shifted rhythmically between her internal and external lives, depending on where we sensed more momentum or need. In the first session I tried to get some information on her history and current situation, much of which I have described above, in order to make these collaborative decisions regarding how best to proceed.

The second and third sessions were emotional for Nina, as we both became acquainted with some of her internal family members. Through a combination of IFS techniques, we were able to meet some of the key players. Over the course of the therapy we worked with nine of her parts, four of which were identified in the second session.

Session 2

Early in the second session, I explained to Nina that I found it useful to view everyone (including myself) as containing any number of subpersonalities or parts, and that our goal would be to get her parts to work together rather than in opposition. If she had balked at the term "parts," I would have used any term that felt better to her—"aspects," "feelings," "thoughts"—but she had no trouble with the language or with the idea that she had many different parts. She said she had always felt that way and wondered whether she was crazy; it was a relief to hear that everyone had them.

Usually it is important to make a statement that normalizes multiplicity to clients before exploring their internal families. Otherwise they are likely to worry that they are, or the therapist thinks they are, sick. If a therapist tries to normalize this process after beginning internal family work, clients may think that they are being placated and that the therapist really thinks they are crazy.

Nina was frantic and tearful about her bulimia, so I began by helping her identify the part of her that was so upset. As I have noted in Chapter 5, when working with a client's internal family, I typically begin by focusing on the protective and managerial parts whose permission I need to enter the system. Nina, however, had been overcome by (blended with) one of her scared, vulnerable parts, and at that point had little access to her managers or to her Self. When a client enters therapy with an exile in the lead, I first work with that part enough to help her separate from it.

I asked Nina to focus on that frantic feeling and put it in a room by itself. Soon after closing her eyes, Nina said that she saw a young girl, maybe 6 or 7 years old, who was crying. As she described this Little Girl, Nina began to calm down and said that she could feel separate from this part.

Many clients will not show this kind of vulnerable, scared part in an early session; instead, they will enter with a manager in the lead. In that state, they may just want to talk about their lives and size me up as we talk. Or they may be reluctant to talk and will give only short responses to my questions. It may be several sessions before I bring up the notion of parts and begin to negotiate with their managers directly. And then it may be many more sessions before these managers have enough trust to give me or the clients access to any exiles.

Most bulimic clients, however, have sporadic episodes in which the hurt or scared parts break out of exile and take over, as they did with Nina prior to our second session. This is terribly distressing to the managers, because they fear the consequences of such vulnerability. With such a client, I work first with these exiles, getting them to separate from the client's Self and helping the Self calm them. When this process is successful, the client's managers are relieved that the client is out of danger, and grateful to the therapist for helping to restore order. Thus, the general rule is that when managers are in control, it is important to get their permission and confidence before working with exiles. When an exile has taken over, the therapist already has access to it, so the therapist can earn credibility with the managers by calming the part, differentiating it from the client's Self, and in essence returning it temporarily to exile. It often feels cold-blooded and counterintuitive not to continue to help a hurt, scared child. But if the exiled part is assured that it will soon be retrieved—this time with the cooperation of the managers, so that it will not have to fight its way out—it can be quite patient. In addition, the consequences can be dire (e.g., retreat from therapy, self-punishing behaviors) if the therapist continues to work with an exile before getting permission from managers.

I asked Nina to let me talk to the Little Girl directly by letting her voice come out of Nina's mouth, as if Nina were sitting in another chair in the office. I chose to talk directly to the part (a method called direct access) instead of having Nina focus inside and interact with the Little Girl herself (a method called in-sight—both direct access and in-sight are described in Chapters 4 and 5), because the Little Girl might have felt as though we were abandoning her if I had immediately asked her to separate from Nina, which would be necessary in order to use in-sight. Through direct access, I could allow her to get to know me and hear that we were going to help her. The Little Girl told me that she was terrified by all kinds of things, but lately she was afraid that Nina was ruining her health with the vomiting. She also feared that she would be lonely forever, because Nina would never get close to anyone again. The Little Girl liked to have fun, but could only do that when she felt secure; consequently, she missed being able to play with and depend on Tom.

Nina's managers kept the Little Girl locked up, because whenever she took over, Nina became scared, needy, and open to being hurt. Indeed, this was the state in which Nina began the second session. The Little Girl interpreted her exile as rejection and abandonment by Nina, which were her two worst fears. She just wanted to be loved by someone; since Nina had rejected her, she seized any opportunity to take over so as to find someone outside of Nina. She knew that what she did to Nina when she blended with her was not good, and she felt guilty for doing it, but she was so overwhelmingly lonely and scared that she could not help it. She wished that she could disappear out of Nina so that she would not cause so much trouble.

When I asked the Little Girl whether she would like Nina to take care of her rather than getting sad with her or scapegoating her, she said that she did not believe Nina wanted to take care of her, or could even if she wanted to. I told the Little Girl that I knew Nina could take care of her and that we would work to get that to happen. I promised to work with the managers to release her from exile, and asked her to wait and not try to take over until we could come and get her. The Little Girl seemed skeptical, but said she would try. I told her that it would probably take some time before Nina's managers developed enough trust to let Nina take care of her. I said I hoped she could be patient.

Before trying to get Nina to help the Little Girl, I wanted to join with the parts that were likely to interfere in that process. When a client begins to try to nurture an exiled part, it is important that she experience success; otherwise, all parts involved will be disappointed and more reluctant to try again. Thus, identifying and negotiating with various managers and firefighters before trying to get close to an exiled part is often a crucial step. After the Little Girl agreed to separate, I asked Nina to identify other parts that reacted strongly to my conversation with the Little Girl. By tracking down the voices she heard or feelings she felt as I talked to the Little Girl, Nina identified three other parts.

The first of these she called Superwoman, and it appeared to her as that comic book character. Superwoman told Nina to be strong at all times and at any cost. She was the part that was in charge of Nina most of the time, and kept her busy to the point of exhaustion by making her take more and more responsibility at work. She left no room for the Little Girl in Nina's daily life. Superwoman also had Nina lift weights and exercise obsessively to make her physically strong. This was the part that steeled Nina so that she could take care of her mother-in-law without breaking down. Superwoman had no patience for the Little Girl, whom she saw as a weak, indulgent cry-baby who kept Nina from moving on.

Nina was so exhausted by the pace Superwoman set, however, that the Little Girl was able to break through frequently. After an episode of the Little Girl's frantic crying, Superwoman attacked Nina for being weak. Superwoman said that she just wanted Nina to forget about the past and get on with her career, so that Nina could feel secure and competent.

A second voice that reacted to my conversation with the Little Girl belonged to a part that Nina called the Protector; this part looked like a muscular woman in a military guard's uniform. The Protector countered the Little Girl's claim that Nina needed to find someone to take care of her by saying that no one could be trusted—everyone could hurt her. She said that Nina should not get too close to or dependent on anyone. This part tried to keep Nina from taking interpersonal risks of any kind and often resorted to criticizing her abilities or features, in an effort to erode her confidence and keep her safe. The Protector made her withdraw from friends; she also searched for and found fatal flaws in any men who seemed interested in Nina. This part kept her isolated, except for her mother-in-law, since Tom's death. Indeed, when Nina had recently considered going out with a man who had been very persistent, the Protector had successfully invoked the memory of Tom in a last-ditch effort to shame her out of the date.

After discussing this role with the Protector, I asked why she had allowed Nina to open up with me, and at what points she might get jumpy. The Protector said that she knew that Nina was in serious trouble, and had decided to sit back for a while to see what I was like. She was not sure about this parts business, and saw a lot of potential danger in allowing me to muck around much further. I assured the Protector that I would proceed at a pace that she and Nina could handle. I would periodically check with her to see how she thought things were going. I also requested that if the Protector felt I was going too fast or recklessly, she should speak up directly rather than eroding Nina's confidence in me or her Self.

In addition, I reminded the Protector about the agreement I made with the Little Girl about being patient and not overwhelming Nina. The Protector was very skeptical about whether the Little Girl could keep this agreement, and, even if she did, whether she could be helped to change. The Protector saw the Little Girl as the embodiment of fear and neediness, and saw no alternative but to keep her isolated. The idea that the Little Girl would no longer be so desperate and destructive if cared for was a new one. Equally disconcerting to the Protector was the idea that she herself played a role in the Little Girl's neediness and fear by keeping her isolated and abandoned. The Protector would have to think about these ideas.

The final part Nina identified during this second session appeared as a haggard, impassive old lady who looked as if she had given up on life. When extreme, this Old Lady told Nina not to care about anything; nothing mattered, so Nina should do whatever she wanted. The Old Lady told Nina that she could not survive without Tom and that there was no hope of life's getting better, so she might as well binge to feel better, since there was no tomorrow to worry about. If she could get Nina to accept such a nihilistic outlook, then Nina would not expect much from people or life and could numb herself with food.

When the Old Lady's attempts to anesthetize Nina were not working and Nina continued to suffer, as had been the case lately, the Old Lady told her to kill herself as a desperate attempt to end the pain. Nina felt her resistance to this advice waning. As a result, Nina's relationship with the Old Lady was ambivalent; she relied on the Old Lady to relieve her suffering, but feared the extremes to which the Old Lady might take her. The Old Lady said that she wanted Nina's life to be free of pain, but that until Nina stopped setting herself up for disappointment by expecting so much of people (as she had of Tom), the Old Lady had to keep her apathetic.

I asked the Old Lady whether there were parts that were naive and trusted everyone, and set Nina up to be disappointed. The Old Lady said that there was such a part; it was different from the Little Girl, but worked with her. I told the Old Lady that we would try to get to know that over-trusting part. I could understand that until she kept that part from setting up disappointments, the Old Lady and the Protector would have to remain vigilant. I also asked the Old Lady to stop recommending suicide, and she agreed to comply for now.

After I finished speaking to all of these parts, I asked Nina how she had experienced the session. She said that it was interesting to overhear those conversations—to hear from these voices one at a time and to hear what they really wanted, rather than the internal clamoring that she usually experienced. But she also felt a bit overwhelmed by all of this, and needed more reassurance that this did not mean she was like Sybil (the MPD patient made famous by a novel and a TV movie). I told her that her internal system seemed polarized, but not so much as the systems of people labeled as having MPD. Also, the Nina I was currently talking to, which I called her Self, seemed to be in a good position to lead her internal system. I could tell this because, once she was separated somewhat from these parts, she (as her Self) had a good perspective on them and on her life. This demonstrated that her parts had enough trust to give some access to her Self.

Nina said that she still felt the need to improve this situation quickly. I reminded her again that we would proceed as slowly as Superwoman, the Protector, and other managers needed to feel safe. We would have to work with the parts that were pressuring for immediate change, so that we did not move too rapidly. Her parts had some good reasons to make her binge and purge, and before she asked them to stop, we had to address their concerns.

Some strategic therapists consider such statements to be paradoxical restraining techniques, in which a therapist tells a client to go slowly to motivate the client to move faster. Unlike those therapists, I make such restraining statements sincerely and without any ulterior motive, because I believe that managers often do have reasonable concerns that must be addressed before lasting change is possible. It is also important for these parts to have some control over the pace and process of therapy, instead of worrying constantly about what the therapist is going to do next.

To avoid confusion, I now summarize the roles of the parts identified by Nina thus far:

The Little Girl—a scared, sad child in exile who was desperate to find a man to take care of her.

Superwoman—a strong, stoic manager who kept exiles at bay by keeping Nina busy working and exercising.

The Protector—a passive, pessimistic manager who kept Nina safe by finding flaws in her or in anyone she got close to and making her withdraw.

The Old Lady—a nihilistic, impulsive firefighter who urged Nina to binge or, at times, to attempt suicide.

Session 3

In the third session we continued identifying the parts that were involved in Nina's bulimia, and clarifying their relationships to one another and to her. Nina came in ready to work. During the week she had tracked down the overly trusting part that the Old Lady had referred to; it was a teenage girl, a "flower child" from the 1960s.

In the second session I had primarily used direct access; I had talked to Nina's parts while her Self observed. Again, I had done this because it is often useful for a client's managers to have direct contact with me, during which they can "sniff me out" to see whether I seem safe. During this third session, however, Nina seemed ready to work with her parts herself, so I shifted to in-sight; that is, I had Nina focus on this trusting feeling and ask the part questions as described in Chapters 4 and 5.

Nina spoke to this trusting Flower Child and found that, indeed, she was extremely naive and innocent. She told Nina that life was supposed to be beautiful and that everyone was good. During the session the Flower Child confessed that she was the one who idealized people—put them on pedestals—so Nina would depend on them. The Flower Child had done this with Tom and hoped to do this now with other men. But the Old Lady and the Protector were preventing her from having much access to Nina.

This pattern was already apparent in our relationship. At times Nina related to me as if she was deeply grateful just to be in my presence, whereas at other times she was wary and guarded. I asked Nina to discuss with the Flower Child whether I had become a target of this part's idealizing, and, if so, why.

The Flower Child acknowledged that this was the case. She recognized that she raised others to such a high level that they could never live up to those unrealistic expectations, and that this elevating kept Nina feeling inadequate. But she believed she had to paint such extremely optimistic pictures of people to counter the hopelessly pessimistic ones the Old Lady and the Protector painted. The Flower Child and the Little Girl worked together to try to get Nina involved with a man. They were the parts that made her feel so wonderful during such relationships.

The Flower Child also admitted that during this period of isolation, while she and the Little Girl were so frustrated and lonely, she gave Nina the urge to binge to fill the emptiness they felt. In this one area she collaborated with the Old Lady, the part that contributed the apathy required to override Nina's concerns about her weight and general appearance.

I asked Nina to find the part that was so concerned about her weight, and she responded that it was *her*, not a part. As much as possible, I try to avoid imposing my preconceptions about a client's internal system on the client. Sometimes, however, a client is so close to or identified with some parts that he or she may not be able to distinguish them from the Self. A client may also have trouble identifying parts who are extremely distant or disengaged from the Self. When I suspect this to be the case, I may ask the client to pretend that such a part exists and act like the part for a few minutes. Or I may simply insist that the part exists and encourage the client to find it. If he or she cannot, it usually means that the part is not ready to expose itself for some reason; for example, it may fear that it will lose power or will be criticized if it comes forth. In that case, I will move on, but remark that I hope the part will feel safe enough to come out sometime in the near future. If the therapist remembers that, by definition, any extreme feelings or thoughts do not characterize the Self, then it is easier to know when one of these hidden parts is operating.

I asked Nina to pretend to be the part that was so concerned about her appearance, and, indeed, the part came to life. Nina called this part the Barbie Doll, because that was what it looked like to her. The Barbie Doll said that she wanted Nina to look perfect so that Nina would attract a man to take care of her. Like several of the others, this appearance-oriented part inherited the burden of patriarchy from Nina's family. She thought that Nina, and women in general, were nothing without the approval and care of men. The Barbie Doll believed that Nina's appearance was all she had to offer a man, so she had to look better than others who had more going for them. This part made Nina diet and constantly criticized the way she looked or presented herself. The Barbie Doll was terrified that all the stress of the last year would make Nina's weight blow up to gigantic proportions. She also hated the parts that were making Nina binge, and she made Nina vomit to keep calories off Nina's thighs.

The Barbie Doll did not believe that she was extreme. She was upset because she thought she had lost power over Nina, now that Nina could see that she was only a part. Nina assured the Barbie Doll that she *was* extreme, but understandably so, given the way that Nina and women in general were raised. Although the Barbie Doll's approval-seeking advice was sometimes useful to her, Nina said she hoped that the part would keep up with her changes and recognize that she did not need the approval of men so much.

The Barbie Doll expressed concern that if she were to back off at all, Nina would stop caring what anybody thought. She worried that Nina not only would let her appearance go, gaining lots of weight, but also would be irritable with people on whom she had to depend. The Barbie Doll made Nina withdraw from a person whenever her anger reached a point where it might be difficult to contain. This was one reason why she had remained so distant from her family. Nina told the Barbie Doll that she understood she would have to find and calm the angry part before the Barbie Doll would be comfortable with a less extreme or powerful role.

Nina had some trouble identifying an angry part, because she said she rarely felt anger. As she focused on those rare times, an angry part—a male—emerged. He was furious with a number of people, from Nina's parents to Tom and his mother. He was also furious with Nina for having kept him so isolated and for allowing people to walk over her all her life. The angry part wanted to be unleashed on some of those people. But he also remembered that the few times he did take over, everyone was scared (including himself and other parts), because Nina became so enraged. When asked to focus on this part, Nina first saw a monster with a dreadful face; however, when I asked her to separate from other parts that were making her fear her anger, the Monster's face softened, and she saw him as sensitive and misunderstood. The Monster told Nina that he would like to help her assert herself, but that she seemed so afraid of him that he had given up hope.

While Nina spoke to this Monster, she became agitated and reported that there was a chorus of voices trying to interfere. I asked her to find these upset parts, and she said it seemed as if nearly all of the others were organized against this Monster. With time running out in the session, Nina decided to respect the fears of this group and not work much more with the Monster at that point. She told the Monster that she would return when the time was right and help him out of his exile.

Nina's other parts were relieved that she had backed off. I asked her to see what she could learn between sessions about why they were so afraid of the Monster. I also warned her not to be surprised if she had extreme emotional reactions that week. When parts are so afraid, they sometimes try to scare or punish the person for getting close to the feared part. Disturbing dreams are not uncommon, as dreams are one way in which parts communicate when they cannot get through directly. Giving a client this kind of anticipatory warning is prudent whenever a change threatens to upset the inner ecology. The reactions of parts to the threat of change cannot always be specifically predicted, even if the parts are asked about them. If the client is prepared, he or she can try to explore their reactions when they occur, instead of being overwhelmed by them.

Again, I recapitulate the roles of parts Nina had identified up to this point. In addition to the exiled Little Girl, the managerial Superwoman and Protector, and the firefighting Old Lady, the third session introduced the following:

> The Flower Child—an exiled teenager who idealized men in hopes that Nina would depend on one.
> The Barbie Doll—a perfectionistic manager who constantly criticized Nina's appearance to try to make her look pleasing to men.
> The Monster—an exiled angry part who felt ignored and impotent.

By this point in the therapy, not only was I learning the characteristics of each part's individual role, but also their interrelationships were coming into focus. It was clear that the dominating managerial coalition included Superwoman, the Protector, and the Barbie Doll. In different ways, they each tried to keep the Little Girl and the Flower Child in protective exile. In addition, Superwoman disdained the Little Girl for being weak and getting everyone hurt, and the Protector hated the Flower Child's gullibility and overtrusting.

These managers relied on the Old Lady to anesthetize the exiles' pain and loneliness. Yet the Barbie Doll hated the Old Lady's calorie-laden binges, and Superwoman saw bingeing as a disgusting lack of will power. These managers also feared the Old Lady's suicidal impulses and further blamed the exiles for triggering them.

Finally, everyone feared the angry Monster and organized to keep him locked out. The Monster's exile was different from that of the Little Girl and the Flower Child. Whereas they were exiled partly for protective reasons, he was exiled purely because the rest feared his firefighter reactions. In this sense, he was less an exile than a firefighter who had been exiled. He hated the approval-seeking pretentiousness of the Barbie Doll and the passivity of the Protector, and they hated him.

Session 4

We began the fourth session by returning to the Monster. Nina had not learned much from her parts during the week, but neither did she have any of the extreme reactions that we had anticipated. It seemed that after our encounter with the Monster her inner system had shut down, waiting for the session before letting her make any moves. This is not an uncommon reaction after a person finds a part the system fears, and is not a problem if the Self is allowed to function in the presence of the therapist.

Nina put the Monster in a room by himself and remained outside the room with her nervous managers. She asked them to let her enter without them; they could watch from outside the room. They reluctantly agreed, and Nina asked the Monster not to overwhelm her with anger as she approached him. Eventually she was able to sit next to him and ask what he was afraid would happen if he were not so angry. After complaining about the passivity of her managers, he admitted that he protected another little girl, and she stepped out from behind him. She was younger than the Little Girl, maybe 4 or 5 years old, and would not raise her head to look at Nina. The Monster agreed that he would not have to remain so angry if this girl were not so vulnerable, and gave permission for Nina to try to help her.

This girl, whom Nina began calling the Scared One, recoiled when Nina first approached her. It took some time and patience before the Scared One would even face Nina, much less speak to her. Eventually she sat on Nina's lap and seemed to enjoy the attention, but also seemed afraid to show her enjoyment. I asked Nina whether she was ready to see where this girl was stuck in the past, and immediately she lost all ability to see anything inside. I asked her to find the part that had turned out the lights; she found the Protector, who was certain that Nina was not ready to see this. After some negotiating, Nina convinced the Protector to allow us to proceed, with the caveat that the Protector could stop the action again at any point she sensed danger.

Nina returned to the Scared One and asked her to show whatever she wanted to about where she was stuck. She first showed a scene during Tom's gradual physical decline. She felt frantic at the prospect of being left alone and ashamed that she could not help him; she thought it was her fault that he was sick. Nina asked whether she was stuck anywhere else, and suddenly Nina could see herself at age 4 in the house where she grew up. Her mother was crying, and her father was telling Nina that it was her fault—that she had been a bad girl. The child was not sure what she had done, but felt totally worthless and responsible. I asked Nina to enter both scenes and be with this Scared One in the way she wished someone had been with her at those times. After Nina held and comforted the girl, she was ready to leave both places and returned to the present with Nina. Nina took her to a pleasant room where the Little Girl and the Flower Child had been staying. Nina then asked the Scared One to find and unload any burdens she carried as a result of those experiences. The Scared One found her sense of worthlessness, which was a sticky black oil covering her hands and arms. When she tried to take it off, however, it quickly returned. I asked Nina to find any parts afraid to let this child unburden her worthlessness. Once again the Protector emerged, complaining that without this worthlessness she would be less able to make Nina withdraw, and that would be risky.

I asked Nina to work with the Protector, and Nina retrieved her from a scene involving her father's rejection at age 10 or 11. Nina helped the Protector see that the father was probably uncomfortable with her budding sexuality and no longer knew how to relate to her. When asked where she carried the burden of protection and fear, the Protector took off the military uniform and revealed herself to be an 11-year-old girl who had been acting older and stronger than she was.

Nina then returned to the Scared One who now was able to wash off the sticky, black substance and felt much relieved without it. She also removed a burden of fear, which was a burning rock in the Scared One's gut. Nina asked who would be willing to look after the Scared One and the Little Girl during the week. The Old Lady volunteered, but the girls were afraid of her. Nina told the Old Lady that we would work with her the next session; until then, Nina would stay with the girls.

Session 5

The fifth session was spent retrieving from the past and unburdening the other parts, beginning with the Old Lady. She carried the burden of hopelessness and was stuck both during Tom's illness and during Nina's adolescence, when it felt as though her whole family were scapegoating her for her rebelliousness. The Monster was next. After Nina's work with the Scared One, he was less angry and less frightening to the others. He was frozen at a time when Nina was a child and her mother was screaming at her father. Nina was terrified, but nonetheless tried to defend her father, shifting her mother's rage onto herself. She carried the burden of her father's rage and the need to protect him. The Monster's retrieval and unburdening transformed him into a feisty teenage boy; he was sensitive to people who might be exploitive, but also loved to exercise and play sports. In a similar process, the Little Girl and the Flower Child were retrieved during the session. They were frozen at the time of Tom's death, as well as at the times of other childhood losses and rejections.

With the retrievals, the parts left the extreme roles they had been forced into and showed who they really were. As they changed, their original names no longer fit, and Nina changed their names. To avoid confusion, however, I continue to use their original names here.

Toward the end of the session, after all these retrievals, Nina seemed distant from me—as if she had lost some trust. I asked about this, and Nina asked inside. She found that Superwoman was feeling more protective, since all these vulnerable parts were now living in the present, where they could be hurt. All this retrieving had made the job of keeping Nina from being hurt more difficult. Nina told Superwoman that although it was true that the parts could be hurt more easily now, they could also be helped more easily if they were hurt, because Nina had access to them. Superwoman was unconvinced, and Nina and I decided to respect her need for distance.

This protective reaction following retrievals is not uncommon and is understandable. The system does feel more vulnerable. It is a mistake for a therapist to misinterpret this reaction as a setback or lack of appreciation. Instead, the therapist should be patient and respectful, but should also encourage the managers to voice their fears.

Session 6

Nina had worked with Superwoman during the week, and wound up retrieving her and the Barbie Doll on her own. They seemed relaxed and out of their extreme roles.

After having done so much internal work, Nina brought up an issue that directed our focus to her external life. Her mother-in-law had again been pressing Nina to visit Tom's grave with her. The prospect of doing so or of refusing again had activated several of Nina's parts. Superwoman and the Old Lady were adamantly against the visit; Superwoman feared Nina would break down at the sight of the grave, and the Old Lady was generally against anything that would activate the Little Girl. On the other hand, several parts, including the Flower Child, the Barbie Doll, and the Little Girl, were afraid to deny a request made by the one significant person in Nina's current life. Nina had decided to go and to try her best to be strong.

I asked Nina to imagine that she was at the graveyard with her mother-in-law and to describe her thoughts and actions. She said that her mother-in-law was telling her stories about Tom between fits of sobbing. Superwoman had taken control of Nina and was giving the tearful woman platitudes, with barely concealed impatience and discomfort. She felt distant from her mother-in-law and knew that she was not being very helpful, but believed she had to rely on Superwoman to keep her from falling apart in that context.

I told Nina to talk with Superwoman and the other activated parts about letting her be her Self with her mother-in-law. They were to try not to interfere, and instead see how it went with Nina's Self in the lead. The parts reluctantly agreed to watch instead of jumping in; Nina then imagined the scene at the cemetery again, but this time with the parts watching in the background instead of struggling to be in control. Nina was amazed at how much more cooperative her parts were after she and they had done the internal work.

After a few minutes of silence, Nina reported that things had gone much better for both women. Nina and her mother-in-law had cried together, holding and stroking each other in commiseration. She felt closer than she ever had to the older woman, and was extremely relieved not to have to pretend to be so strong. I asked Nina how her parts reacted to this; she said that they seemed impressed and surprised that it went so well, although Superwoman was still skeptical. Nina decided to try to repeat this experiment *in vivo* that week, and I wished her luck.

I find that this kind of in-sight (which I call the "Self-confidence technique") is often useful for helping a client's parts see that they can trust the Self. When parts let the Self lead in external situations, those situations are inevitably handled better than when a part leads. If parts refuse to allow the Self to lead, then their fears can be explored and addressed until they are willing to temporarily cede control to the Self.

Session 7

At the seventh session, Nina proudly reported that her trip to the cemetery had unfolded almost as she had envisioned: She and her mother-in-law were able to cry together. She was also surprised at how nurturing her mother-in-law was able to be, once Nina gave her the chance. The Little Girl, in particular, felt relieved by finally being able to share her sorrow with someone and to be free of Superwoman's stranglehold. Superwoman was duly impressed and was also relieved not to have to maintain the strong front constantly. I asked Nina to bring Superwoman and the Little Girl together, to talk about how they might want to reorganize their relationship. With some encouragement from Nina, the Little Girl was able to say how much she admired Superwoman and would like to spend time with her. Superwoman was remarkably happy to do this, and Nina agreed to monitor this change in their relationship.

By this point, Nina's bingeing and purging had abated considerably. The Little Girl felt less desperate now that Nina's mother-in-law had become a source of support instead of a burden. Nina knew, however, that her parts were still polarized in certain areas, especially her relationships with men. Since Superwoman had begun to relax, the Flower Child and Little Girl had become more vocal about finding a man. Predictably, this activated the Protector and the Old Lady to counter such urges, and the Barbie Doll to focus on the inadequacies of Nina's appearance.

Since Nina worked in a health club, she was often around men, many of whom asked her out. Soon after Tom's death, the Flower Child had overridden the concerns of other parts and created an unrealistically positive picture of one of these men. He had seemed strong and able to be sensitive. Nina had gone out with him several times, opening her tortured heart with the expectation that his apparent empathy and strength could help her heal. He was frightened by her vulnerability and ended their relationship abruptly and coldly. The Protector and Old Lady seized that incident as confirmation of their views of men, and of Nina's poor judgment regarding them; subsequently, they refused to let her near a man. In re-examining that relationship, Nina was able to see that although this man may not have been the best choice at that time, the extremes of her Flower Child probably contributed to his behavior. She concluded that if she were ever to develop a supportive relationship with a man, the Flower Child needed to feel herself a valuable part of the inner group, in addition to having been retrieved and unburdened.

Session 8

Nina began the eighth session by summoning all the parts we had identified into a room while she, as her Self, observed them from outside the room through a window. She saw the Protector and Superwoman together on one side of the room, and the Little Girl, the Scared One and the Old Lady together on the other side. The Flower Child was pacing, the Barbie Doll was standing alone, and the Monster was sitting in a corner watching. None of the parts were interacting; instead, they seemed to be waiting for something to happen. I asked Nina how she was feeling about the whole group and she said she wanted to go in and talk to them.

If while watching her parts Nina had reported any extreme emotions, such as feeling overwhelmed by them or angry at one or another, I would have asked her to find other parts that were influencing her to feel those extreme ways and put them into the room as well. I would not have asked her to address the whole group until she felt ready to lead. She said she wanted to help the parts resolve their issues regarding men.

Nina said that her parts looked at her expectantly as she entered the room, and responded when she told them to come and sit in front of her. She asked to speak to the parts that were most upset about the idea of her beginning to date. After some discussion among them it was determined that the Flower Child and the Protector were the most polarized. Nina had these two come forward and sit facing each other while the others watched. She asked them to talk with each other directly, while she played the role of their therapist.

Initially, the Protector displayed intense scorn, almost hatred, for the Flower Child, who was intimidated and reluctant to talk. With some suggestions from me, Nina skillfully and firmly insisted that they talk to each other about their relationship and do so in a respectful manner. The tone of their conversation shifted surprisingly quickly. The Flower Child apologized for putting Nina in jeopardy with the last man. In turn, the Protector said that she knew the Flower Child had Nina's best interests at heart, but the Flower Child had to understand that other parts were very vulnerable and so Nina had to be careful. They agreed that the Protector would lift the moratorium on dating if the Flower Child promised not to try to take over and make Nina rush into a position of dependence or vulnerability.

Nina was amazed with the ease at which this agreement between former mortal enemies was reached. I reminded her that their ability to make such deals so easily was, in large part, the result of her increased leadership. That is, both parts were able to lay down their burdens and make concessions, because each believed that Nina would hold the other to the deal. In the absence of trusted leadership, such deals are impossible. The fact that these parts so readily compromised and respected Nina's directives was a tribute to the work Nina had done in the previous weeks to demonstrate to them that she could lead.

In a similar way, Nina brought forward each of the other parts to discuss their concerns or needs regarding men and to work out their differences. At times Nina was frustrated with the slow pace at which certain parts were participating. In searching for the source of her impatience, she discovered another part lurking in the background, which she called the Daredevil. This part was easily bored and had been chronically frustrated with the lack of excitement in Nina's life. As a result, it kept Nina spinning with a sense of directionless urgency, which interfered with her ability to make and stick to decisions and made her impatient with the pace of any changes. After Nina assured the Daredevil that its desires for fun and excitement would be addressed by the group at another meeting, that part stopped interfering, and the group meeting proceeded more smoothly.

When things seem to bog down in IFS work, it is not uncommon to discover that the impasses are the result of interference from a hidden part. The key to finding such a part is frequently to ask the client how he or she is feeling, and to listen carefully for even slight departures from the compassionate or curious Self. This is particularly true during an impasse.

Ultimately, the group decided that the Protector would monitor the degree to which Nina became dangerously close to any man with whom she went out. But instead of enlisting the Old Lady to help find flaws in the man and make Nina apathetic toward him (as had been the part's style), the Protector would cue the Monster, who would provide advice to Nina as to how to handle the situation in a direct, assertive way. Superwoman would continue to support the Little Girl, and Nina also would visit the Little Girl and Scared One more frequently, so that they would not become extremely needy or vulnerable in the process. In addition, Nina would keep an eye on the Flower Child and the Barbie Doll to make sure they did not take over. Finally, the whole group would meet regularly to consult on the progress with this issue and plan for other issues.

Session 9

At the ninth session Nina was quite pleased with herself. She had eaten normally all week and had not had to fight to do so. She continued to meet with her parts to consolidate plans and changes. Although she had not gone out with anyone because she had had no tempting invitations, she felt confident that when she met an interesting man she would not hesitate. In the meantime, the Daredevil had come up with a series of proposals the group was considering for having fun without a man. In general—with the exception of the Barbie Doll, who still said that men were all-important—the parts were united behind the goal of Nina's renewing her friendships with several women whom she had neglected through all of her travails.

By this session our roles had shifted significantly. Over the previous several sessions, I had moved from directing Nina in how to talk to her parts, to asking her what she thought she needed to do with them. As is true of many clients, her Self was able to take the lead quickly, allowing me to remain in a supportive rather than a directive role much of the time. In this session the shift was even more apparent, because instead of Nina's presenting me with a problem and our struggling together to find a solution, Nina had done most of the work prior to the session and was simply reporting her progress.

Such a shift often represents a consolidation of a client's internal leadership and indicates that the therapist can experiment with a further diminished role. The eagerness and determination with which Nina was working between sessions by this time allowed me to accelerate the shift of responsibility for therapy. We agreed to meet the next week to check on progress, and, if it was maintained, to increase the interval between sessions.

Session 10

At the 10th session, Nina reported that she had continued to meet nightly with her parts, and had focused particularly on her relationship with the Barbie Doll. She disabused that part of the insistent belief that Nina was nothing without a man. Nina did this by following through on her plans to reconnect with women friends and demonstrating that she could enjoy herself and achieve some intimacy in nonromantic relationships. Nina shared her grief with some of these friends and found their outpouring of support both surprising and nurturing. On the basis of this experience, she placed the goal of becoming close to a man lower on her list of priorities, and decided instead to concentrate on these renewed relationships and on her estranged family of origin.

Before I began using the IFS model, I would have directed Nina several sessions earlier not to try to find a man before she had developed a network of friends and had established to herself that she could survive independently. Since developing and using the model, I have come to believe that such a directive at that point would have activated several parts against the directive and against me. I also find that instructions like this one are often unnecessary, because, as in Nina's case, clients frequently make the same decisions that I would have suggested, and at the proper point rather than when I would have wanted the moves made.

Nina also reported that since she was feeling strong, she had entertained the idea of trying to re-enter her family. She had begun preparing for this by envisioning encounters with her mother and father in which she told her parts to stay back and let her Self handle things. Much as when she did this in preparation for the trip to the cemetery with her mother-in-law, in her mind, Nina was able to tell her mother that she felt disappointment with her mother's lack of support during the past several years. In response, her mother described her hurt at what she perceived to be messages from Nina that she did not want her support. This in-sight work gave Nina a new perspective on her interactions with her mother, and made her eager to meet with her mother *in vivo*.

Sessions 11 through 14

We decided to spread out subsequent sessions, since Nina was continuing to make progress on her own. We met again in 2 weeks, and followed that session with three more at 2-week intervals. During this 2-month period Nina was increasingly able to work with her internal system on her own. She met with her mother and decided that she did not need to confront her, since she had already done so through in-sight. Instead they slowly warmed to each other. Nina gradually disclosed more about her ordeal before, during, and after Tom's death, and her mother spoke of how much she wished she had been able to help but had felt shut out.

The Monster helped Nina approach this meeting from a strong position by reminding her that she could now function on her own. As a result, Nina felt less vulnerable to rejection and more able to express differences without fear of further reprisals. From this position, she could be with her parents and siblings without becoming part of the sequences of interaction that had driven her out earlier.

After the 14th session, Nina's progress seemed solid. She was finding that she had to do less direct work with her parts because they seemed to be cooperating spontaneously, as if each now respected her leadership and had evolved into a new, nonextreme role within the system. Certain parts still became extreme periodically, particularly the Old Lady and the Little Girl, but Nina found that she could usually calm them quickly; on the rare occasions when she was unable to calm them, she no longer believed the extreme things they said and could remain her Self while they were extreme. Thus, her parts were no longer triggering the internal sequences that led to binge–purge episodes. By the 14th session, Nina had been eating normally for about 3 months. We agreed that she was ready to prove to herself that she could maintain this without my help, and we terminated the sessions with the proviso that she could return at any point she deemed necessary.

Follow-up

About 9 months later, Nina asked for another session. She had been doing well, although several parts had become extreme at various times, particularly around the anniversary of her husband's death. In general, she still was able to calm or control the parts when they became activated; she had had no further bulimic episodes; and her external relationships had continued to improve. She returned to see me because she had allowed herself to become involved with a man, Don, and was struggling with the parts that this aroused.

As I listened to Nina discuss the issue with her group of parts, it became clear that although the Protector and the Old Lady were activated, they were not as fervent or caustic as before. Instead, they expressed their legitimate concerns directly and clearly. Similarly, the Flower Child and the Little Girl, while still highly desirous of a relationship with a man, were willing to consider that this might not be the relationship for Nina.

It appeared that Don had some extreme parts of his own. He adored Nina to the point of wanting to be with her all the time. He reacted strongly to any sign that Nina was not totally available to him, including her anniversary reaction to her husband's death. He was already talking of marriage. Nina was afraid that out of fear of being overwhelmed by his urgency, she would break off all contact with him. The Protector and the Old Lady were pressing for immediate withdrawal, which had been their previous pattern when men had been interested. Nina wanted to tell Don that he needed to back off, and the Monster thought that he could help her do that, but she did not trust that she could do so without making Don feel bad.

I helped Nina negotiate a plan with her group of parts; then, through in-sight, she had the conversation with Don as her Self, while her parts watched. Later the *in vivo* conversation with him went as well as it had through in-sight, yet Nina's protective parts still had grave reservations about him. Nina decided to remain in the relationship, if for no other reason than to work with these parts on trusting her to care for the system, no matter what Don did.

Don began working with another IFS therapist, who helped him comfort his exiles so that he could be less possessive. As Nina saw Don struggle with rather than deny his vulnerability, her Monster, Old Lady, and Protector gradually joined to support him instead of attacking his denial. Don and Nina are now married, and for the 4 years since our initial therapy, bulimia has not been a problem for Nina.

Discussion

This case exemplifies the course and outcome of using the IFS model with many clients. Many people are like Nina in their ability to do much of the work on their own, once they get to know some parts and differentiate their Selves. For some clients, however, IFS therapy involves many more sessions and is more intense. Often, such a client has been hurt, scared, or betrayed more severely than Nina, so the parts have less trust in me or in the Self. For example, whereas Nina's parts generally cooperated when she asked them to separate, this would not be the case with someone whose inner family was more polarized and distrusting. Whereas Nina's managers allowed me entrance to her inner system relatively quickly, with other clients I have to spend many sessions working with managers before they trust that it is safe. In fact, with some clients (usually survivors of severe abuse), IFS therapy can take several years and at times can seem very slow (Goulding & Schwartz, in press).

When the process does not move as quickly or smoothly as it did with Nina, it is not always because of the client's internal family. The client may live in a constraining external family or environment. Or parts of the therapist may be interfering; this is particularly true when the therapist is new to the IFS work and is uncertain about how things will go. The client may sense the therapist's insecurity and, understandably, may keep the doors closed.

The point of all this is that internal systems have their own pace and wisdom. I have learned to respect that pace and not to prejudge how much time or how many sessions a client will need. I have also learned to work with parts of me before, during, and after sessions that might interfere with the work with a particular client.

The work with Nina also illustrates another important point. Even after many of her parts had been depolarized, unburdened, and retrieved, they sometimes reverted to their extreme roles in the face of new activation, such as the idea of getting close to a man. This is not uncommon, and some therapists mistake it as evidence of relapse. Instead, it is a natural tendency for parts to return temporarily to what they perceived as safe or familiar roles and burdens in the face of a threat. The difference is that once a part has been retrieved and unburdened, it can quickly leave its extreme role, once it is reminded that the role is not needed.

As complex as this therapy with Nina may seem, we had a big advantage because she was independent and not caught up in constantly activating external relationships. When this is not the case, the therapist must understand and work with a larger network of people and their parts. Chapters 6, 7, and 8 provide guidelines for that work.

CHAPTER 4

Changing
the Internal System

Chapter 2 has presented the conceptual side of the IFS model as it applies to individuals and Chapter 3 illustrated the process of IFS therapy. The next two chapters describe the IFS methods used with Nina in Chapter 3. This much attention is devoted to work with individuals not because the intrapsychic is the most important system level, but because once a therapist can understand and apply the model at this level, it is easier to use it at family or cultural levels.

This chapter provides an overview of the process—describing goals, guidelines, and warnings for the specific steps therapist and client take together during this adventure. Chapter 5 describes the different modes for accessing and working with a person's internal family.

The Therapist–Client Relationship

The Therapist's Assumptions

The way a therapist relates to a client is strongly related to whether or not the therapist believes that people have within them the ability to deal effectively with their problems. If so, the therapist will work with clients to discover and change whatever is constraining them from exercising those abilities. If, on the other hand, the therapist believes that people have problems because they lack something—whether that something is a strong enough ego, adequate information about the problem, a workable view of it, medication, or a nurturing parent or mate—then the therapist will try to give clients what they lack (whether through reparenting, interpretations, information, reframes, directives, or drugs). The primary difference I am highlighting here is the difference between a collaborative partnership in which people are given the message that they have what it takes, and an authoritative relationship implicit in which is the message that clients are somehow lacking or defective.

In the reality of clinical practice, therapists will vacillate between these two positions. The collaborative therapist will sometimes give information, sympathy, or directives, and the authoritative therapist will sometimes encourage clients to use their own resources. The difference, then, is not so much in the therapist's behavior, but instead in his or her overall attitude toward clients and the messages that this attitude conveys.

The IFS model suggests that everyone has a Self that, once differentiated, can balance and harmonize the internal system. When a client is not able to do this, the therapist assumes that the client's Self is constrained by imbalances in the surrounding systems. The goal of therapy becomes to help the client identify and change the internal and external constraints that are preventing Self-leadership. Thus, the therapist's job is to try to help the client differentiate qualities that allow the client to understand and change his or her predicaments. IFS presumes that those qualities exist in the client, and the therapist's job is to help the client elicit them.

Hermann Hesse (1927/1975) once wrote, "I wanted only to try to live in accord with my true Self. Why was that so very difficult?" The IFS model helps people find and change the things that are making it difficult.

Collaboration

These positive assumptions about people allow for a highly collaborative therapist–client relationship. The therapist trusts that if released from their constraints, clients have the ability to see their predicaments in useful ways and to act effectively; thus, the therapist does not have to provide clients with interpretations, reframes, or directives about their symptoms. When a client's Self is in the lead, the client will be able to discover from the parts why they do extreme things and what needs to change internally. When the client's family members' Selves are in the lead, they will be able to identify the patterns or parts that constrain the client, and what needs to change in these external family relationships. The therapist, by asking questions and by conveying the IFS assumptions and techniques, creates a context in which people are freed from the internal and external polarizations that constrain them from doing these things for themselves.

Thus, the therapist joins the client (and, when appropriate, the client's family) in a collaborative effort to identify and change internal and external constraints to the client's Self-leadership. The therapist brings to clients these empowering IFS assumptions: Everyone has parts that are valuable but are in constraining roles, and everyone has, at the core, a Self with wonderful leadership qualities. Otherwise, the therapist becomes a curious, empathic, and respectful partner to clients. Initially, the therapist may take more of a leadership role by asking questions about certain kinds of constraints and by suggesting ways to differentiate a client's Self so that the client can deal with the constraints. Even when making suggestions or leading people through parts work, however, the therapist solicits and respects the client's ideas about these interventions and about his or her experience. As a client's Self emerges and takes more initiative, the therapist can and should quickly share this leadership, so that therapy feels like a genuine partnership.

Thus, primary responsibility for creating change is not placed on the therapist, as it is in some family therapies, or on the client, as it is in some psychoanalytic therapies. Instead, in the IFS model, responsibility is shared between client and therapist. It is as if the therapist's and the client's Selves are cotherapists, working together to harmonize the client's parts and external world. When a client's Self is unavailable for an extended period (as is sometimes the case with survivors of severe childhood sexual abuse), the therapist may temporarily act as a unilateral leader until the client's parts trust the therapist's Self and the client's Self enough to step back and let the client's Self lead. In that case, the cotherapy relationship between the client's and therapist's Selves develops more gradually.

When such cotherapy partnerships are established, clients often do much of the internal work between sessions, both following through on plans devised in a session and exploring further on their own. This ability of clients to do much of the work outside the therapist's office makes the therapy briefer and more empowering for the clients, and more enjoyable for the therapist, than therapies in which clients are more dependent on the therapist's insights or direction.

Therapist's Parts

For therapist's to maintain such collaborative attitudes and relationships, they must, as much as possible, lead with their own Selves and keep their own extreme parts from interfering. Thus, therapists need to be aware of some of their own parts that are activated by the practice of psychotherapy generally, and by certain types of clients or problems in particular. Therapists need to monitor these parts and find ways to keep them from taking over through the course of therapy. This does not necessarily require that a therapist receive therapy, because many people can achieve enough Self-leadership on their own to be effective clinicians. It can help a great deal, however, to sit down with someone periodically and work on one's own internal system. Those therapists who are the most effective with this model are those who understand it intuitively because they know their own internal families.

Parts of therapists that commonly interfere with providing effective therapy include the following:

- Striving managers that become critical if change isn't rapid enough, can become highly directive or coercive, and cannot stand to be in the presence of weakness or vulnerability: "You have to tell her what's going on; she's too overwhelmed to ever understand." "He's been coming to see you for over a year—some brief therapist you are." "All she does is cry—why can't she quit sniveling and just move on?"

- Approval-seeking managers that often want clients to depend on or worship a therapist, or worry about not being liked or seen as effective if clients are displeased or upset: "Now you made her mad at you and she won't like you and will tell everyone that you and your stupid model are no good."

- Pessimistic managers that, when things are not going well, might tell a therapist to give up or blame clients: "He's much sicker than you thought." "You don't know what you're doing." "She's always trying to manipulate you, so who cares about her pain?"

- Caregiving managers that may want to take over for clients, or can't stand for clients to be upset, or need to rescue them: "You have to do it for him—he's obviously incapable." "You are bad if you ever let her suffer."

- Angry parts that can make the therapist impatient with clients and feel burdened by them: "What does he want now? It's always some big crisis." "She's so dependent, so demanding—why can't she just be strong?" "Maybe he'll cancel this week."

- Hurt parts that overidentify with clients' pain: "How could he stand that? That was too horrible! Don't listen, it's too much!" "She can't take any more—you've got to do something, or get her to, to stop it now!" "It's too much like your own pain that you try to stay away from."

- Evaluating parts that are critical of the therapist's own weight, eating habits, relationships, or general indulgences, and also can't stand those things in others: "My God, she's thinner than you and she's complaining—you must really be a pig!"

A therapist needs to be aware of when these and other parts interfere during sessions. He or she must be able either to get those parts to step back and trust the Self, or, when that is not possible, to acknowledge to the client that a part is interfering and apologize for it. The therapist need not and cannot always be a model of Self-leadership, but he or she can model taking responsibility for times when parts interfere and trying to prevent that. My colleagues and I have an axiom: "When you encounter a problem in IFS therapy, it is usually because a part is interfering, but you don't know whose it is—the client's or yours."

Transference and Countertransference

Sometimes the reason why a part interferes is that it is frozen in the past and relates to the situation from that perspective. This is similar to what is known as "transference" and "countertransference" in psychodynamic models. Although it is not uncommon for clients to relate to me as if I were someone from their past (transference), and I may view a client at times in the same way I viewed one of my parents (countertransference), the IFS model understands and treats this phenomenon somewhat differently. It is not a client who is seeing me as a parent or abuser or sibling. It is just a part of him or her that sees me that way—a part that is frozen in the past at an emotionally laden time, or a part that carries a burden from interactions with the original person.

If, for example, a female client has an exiled child part that is frozen at a point where she was repeatedly rejected by her father, that part may be desperate for my approval, and another protector part, expecting that I also will reject her, will be constantly pushing me away and seeing me as untrustworthy. Although it is possible for me to discuss this transference in the context of our current relationship, it is also possible for me to ask the client to find the parts that have these transferred feelings or beliefs, and to help her retrieve or unburden those parts (as described in this and the next chapter). After being released from their burdens or from the point in time in which they are stuck, parts no longer hold these anachronistic views or emotions.

The exceptions to this are the small percentage of my clients whose abuse was so severe and chronic that their Selves are temporarily inaccessible. Their protective managers will not allow their Selves to lead, so I relate directly to their parts. As a result, I encounter directly their distorted perceptions of me. These are often particularly challenging relationships because I am exposed to all types of provocation, accusation, or expectation. It helps to remember that only a part of such a client has temporarily taken over and is relating to me this way—a part that is frozen at a time when there were good reasons to relate to authority figures in these extreme ways. If I can maintain Self-leadership in the face of such activation, gradually the part will realize that I am different from the person it has me confused with. I then will be allowed to retrieve and unburden it.

Therapists who are successful in maintaining some degree of Self-leadership will, by definition, feel and express curiosity and compassion for their clients' predicaments and respect for the clients' abilities. This does not mean that the therapist will not feel other emotions, such as anger, happiness, or sadness. Their parts are not banished; they will be there to advise and color their experience. The feedback that therapists' parts provide clients, when these parts are not extreme, can be invaluable, and therapists are encouraged to give reports from their parts to clients. Before speaking for a part, however, a therapist must try to determine whether the part is extreme and distorting in its perceptions; if unsure as to whether it is, he or she should report this uncertainty to the client. It is therapists' responsibility to work with their own parts outside of sessions, to keep them from distorting and interfering, and to maintain the compassion and respect of Self-leadership.

This compassion and respect will be conveyed consistently through tone of voice and nonverbal behavior. Thus, therapists who are leading with their Selves will, if necessary, be able to say things that in content are challenging of clients, yet will still convey an underlying sense of compassion and respect. When this is the case, clients will not respond so defensively, because they will hear the caring along with the criticism. Their Selves will be elicited by their therapists' Selves.

It is often difficult, however, for therapists to maintain this kind of compassionate Self-leadership. With many clients, therapy is a rollercoaster, full of sudden drops. A therapist who is highly invested in rapidly alleviating symptoms will feel happy when a client is doing well and discouraged, defensive, and pessimistic when he or she is not, which will feed the client's unproductive pessimism and inner recrimination. Similarly, the therapist may have difficulty maintaining Self-leadership in the face of angry or distancing parts of the client or family members that try to protect them from harm by not trusting anyone. Or, if the client's family members are angry or disdainful toward the therapist, the therapist may have trouble not disliking them and trying to protect himself or herself from them.

If instead the therapist can remain steady, curious, and confident through the troubled waters—can remain the "I in the storm"—then the client and family members can regain their Self-leadership rather than falling into vicious cycles of despair or anger. The therapist and client can calmly explore what provoked the setback and take steps to repair and prevent it. They can learn from rather than fall victim to apparent relapses.

These are but a few examples of potential mines in the minefield that IFS therapy can be. A therapist who can maintain Self-leadership will be able to express what might be called "tenacious caring"—caring in the face of sometimes constant provocation—and the therapy will succeed. The nice thing about this kind of work is that the rewards for the therapist's internal system are often as great as for the client's. The struggle to maintain Self-leadership is extremely therapeutic.

Introducing the Language

The language of the IFS model, in and of itself, is quite relieving and empowering for clients. Once they discover that their rage, shame, incompetence, or neediness come not from their basic personalities but from little parts of them—parts that they can help change—then life doesn't seem so bleak. They realize that there is much more to them than these extreme parts, and that these other resources can be brought to bear to help these parts.

The first steps toward achieving this goal involve introducing a shift in the way the clients describe themselves and their problems—a shift away from monolithic language to the language of multiplicity. For most clients, this shift is remarkably easy and is welcomed. Most people seem to believe this about themselves already, or at least to have an intuition about it, and sometimes spontaneously use the language (e.g., "A part of me wants to go to the reunion, but another part is afraid to").

One way to introduce the language is to have clients describe their problems or how they are feeling, and then feed back to them what they said, but in the parts language. Here is an example:

MARY: I try to do better at not purging, and sometimes I succeed, but my parents only see that I'm still doing it—they don't see my progress—and that takes away the thought of "Boy, I'm doing well."

THERAPIST: It makes you not want to try any more?

MARY: Yeah. I know that I'm doing better, but still I also feel like "Well, why bother?" It's almost an excuse, because then I think I may as well do it, but then I think, "No, I should stop."

THERAPIST: It sounds like there are several different parts of you arguing about this. One part is hurt by your parents' lack of recognition and tells you to give up, and another part pushes you to keep trying no matter what they do. Does that sound right?

MARY: Yeah. That's right.

THERAPIST: And what else do you hear in there? Is there a part that criticizes you all the time?

MARY: Yeah, there are many times when I feel like a loser because I can't stop purging.

THERAPIST: So when you purge, this part jumps on your back and calls you a loser?

MARY: (*Sobbing*) Yeah.

THERAPIST: That doesn't help, does it? And it looks like there's a part around now that makes you feel kind of sad. Is that right?

MARY: Yeah, it's been around a lot lately.

Mary's last response indicates that she had gone beyond just accepting the language and was beginning to use it. Virtually any statement a client makes can lead to an opening to introduce the language of parts:

MRS. JOHNSON [Mary's mother]: I can't stand the mess she leaves in the bathroom. If she doesn't start taking care of it soon, I don't know what I'm gonna do.

THERAPIST: What do you say to yourself when you find the mess in the bathroom?

MRS. JOHNSON: I say that she's doing this on purpose to bother me—to rub my nose in it.

THERAPIST: How does this part of you that tells you she's doing it to bother you make you act toward Mary?

MRS. JOHNSON: I yell at her then. I threaten to throw her out. Then I feel guilty about that. But I don't know what else to do.

THERAPIST: What do you say to yourself when you feel guilty?

MRS. JOHNSON: I say that I'm a bad mother and it's my fault that she's got this problem in the first place, so I shouldn't be upset with her.

THERAPIST: So there's one part that gets furious with her, and another that argues with it and attacks you. Is that right?

MRS. JOHNSON: Yeah—pretty crazy, right?

THERAPIST: No—a pretty normal reaction to a scary problem. But, even though it's normal, it sounds like this war between these parts gets in the way of you being the way you want to with Mary. Is that right? Would you like to change your relationship with each of those parts?

As illustrated in the second example, the question "What do you say to yourself?" is very useful in accessing inner dialogue. The client responds with "I say _____," and the therapist can then translate with "Oh, so a part of you says _____. Do you ever argue with yourself about this?" The client responds, "Yes, I think _____." The therapist again translates to the client: "Oh, so this part disagrees with the other." The goal at this stage is for the therapist, through this translation process, to introduce the parts language gently to the client, and for both therapist and client to become acquainted with some of the client's parts that play key roles in his or her problems.

Some people initially have trouble with the idea that they are not unitary personalities and will resist using this language. This may be because parts of them fear that they are, or that the therapist thinks they are, crazy or have MPD. Or they may generally be afraid of revealing their inner lives or of being coerced into a particular view of things by the therapist, and pick the language issue as a battleground. Or they may be dominated by a part that will not relinquish power until it has ventilated and knows the therapist understands its perspective: "Don't talk about my parts! It's Mary's messing up my bathroom that is the problem here." Or the therapist feels uneasy using the language; he or she expects that clients will think it's silly or bizarre, and conveys that insecurity to the clients.

Whatever the reason, when I encounter resistance to the parts language, I usually stop using it and wait until it seems that the client trusts me more before introducing it again. When I was insecure about how people would react to it, I encountered much more resistance than I do now. It is quite rare for a client to be uncomfortable when I present the model when my Self is in the lead.

Beginners tend to make one of two mistakes at this point. Either they rush to indoctrinate clients, introducing the parts language too early or with too much vigor and too many words; this often creates defensive reactions in clients, which then lead the therapists to give up completely or to sell even harder. The other mistake is to be so tentative and inconsistent about the language that it never gets established, and the therapists assume that the clients won't relate to it.

At some point after having used the language, I will usually introduce some of the basic ideas of the IFS model. I say something like the following:

You may have noticed me using the term "parts" to describe your feelings or thoughts. I do that because I believe that we all have many different personalities that fight inside and try to take over power from one another. When they are at war, it feels like you are out of control, doesn't it? And sometimes a part will take over and make you do or say things you don't want to do, right? Well, I know that even though those parts of you get extreme and destructive at times, they all want something good for you. I know how to help you get them to change into their preferred roles so they get along with each other and stop doing this to you. Are you interested?

Depending on the degree to which the client's managers trust me at that point, this may be all I need to say to explain what we may do before proceeding. With some clients, I need to discuss the model and the techniques at greater length before their managers relax. As I describe later, I have a great deal of respect for managers and will discuss with them as much as they need to feel more assured.

Discussing Internal Relationships

Once the parts language has been introduced and accepted by clients to some degree, and they have agreed to try to use the model, there are several levels at which the model can be used. Probably the least threatening level is simply to ask the clients questions about their parts and the part's relationship with the client and with one another.

As different parts are identified during discussions of a person's problem, the therapist can ask questions about each part's relationship with the Self, with other parts, or with other people in the external environment. The goal is for both therapist and client to get a sense of the inner ecology that they are entering. It is wise for therapists who are beginning to use the IFS model to spend a lot of time with clients at this stage of talking about parts and their relationships. It is important to have an awareness of key internal relationships in advance of entering a client's system, so that the therapist's and the client's Selves can plan interventions and anticipate reactions. Therapists who are more experienced with the model will often spend less time with clients discussing these internal relationships, because, with an awareness of many common internal patterns, they feel confident entering clients' internal systems relatively quickly to learn about these patterns from the parts themselves or as the clients' Selves describe what the parts tell them. In a case where a client's managers seem extremely fearful or mistrusting, even an experienced therapist will be wise to remain at the level of discussing parts rather than talking to them directly until the managers seem more trusting. Described below are some content areas for this discussion.

Relationship between a Part and the Self

Once a client identifies a part, the therapist can ask how the client feels toward it; why the client thinks it does what it does; how often the client hears from it; how much influence it has over the client, and vice versa; and, in general, how the client would like his or her relationship with it to change. The therapist can ask the client to focus on the identified part between sessions and monitor when, where, and by whom it is activated;

how it affects the client when it is activated; and how well the client can calm it or get it to separate from him or her.

Relationship between Two Parts

The therapist can ask the same questions about the relationship between two parts. That is, how does the client think these two parts feel toward, influence, or activate each other? Why do they relate this way? It is particularly important to explore highly polarized or protective relationships. It can be helpful to ask the client to think about how two polarized parts sabotage each other and how they might be helped to get along better. The therapist may ask the client not only to monitor these parts between sessions, but also to try to talk to each of them about how they don't have to do these extreme things and can trust him or her more than they do.

Highly polarized parts will not become less extreme unilaterally. That is, since each side of the polarization fears that the other will leap to take over if it backs down, each polarized part has to trust that the other will change its role at the same time that it makes a change. For this to occur, each must trust that the Self will not let the other take over. The same is true for highly protective internal relationships. The protective part cannot give up that protective role until it knows that the part it protects will be safe and cared for by the Self.

This bilateral or ecological nature of internal change highlights two important guidelines. First, if a client is trying to get an extreme part to change, he or she should try to find, and include in the change equation, the part or parts that the initial part is polarized with or protects. Second, anything the client can do to increase the parts' trust in the Self will help.

Increasing Trust in the Self through External Work

Because most clients have not had their Selves in the lead, and have been directed in one extreme way or another by warring parts, their parts often have little faith that their Selves can lead. For this reason, some parts of them are oriented toward finding people in the external world to take care of them, while others are equally desperate not to trust such people, for fear of getting hurt.

There are many ways for a client's parts to gain trust in the leadership ability of the Self, and not all of these ways involve internal work. For example, as a client is able to talk to his or her parents about risky subjects with the Self in the lead, the client's parts increasingly see that they don't need to protect him or her so much and that the Self can handle risky situations. Thus, if the therapist is reluctant to enter the internal realm because of a lack of confidence or because he or she thinks the client's Self is not trusted enough, the therapist and client can discuss external situations where the client can experiment with leading with the Self. Much of Bowen's therapy (Bowen, 1978; Kerr & Bowen, 1988), in fact, can be seen as this kind of work. The IFS therapy often alternates between a client's working with his or her internal system and experimenting with Self-leadership in external relationships.

Entering the Internal System Safely

In the IFS model, there are two basic ways of entering and working directly with a client's internal system. One of these is called "direct access." In it, the therapist talks directly to one or more parts, or, using the open-chair technique pioneered by Gestalt therapy, has parts talk directly to one another or to the Self. The other is called "in-sight" and involves having the client look inside to find and work with parts that he or she sees or senses and describes to the therapist. Both of these methods are powerful; consequently, they are dangerous if applied without sufficient knowledge of the potential problems and how to avoid them. Before describing the modalities of direct access and in-sight in Chapter 5, I outline some of the dangers and guidelines here.

Child-Like Exiles

As described in Chapter 2, virtually every client with whom I have used this model has young, child-like parts (when using in-sight, they often appear as children of various ages). When upset, these young parts feel some combination of the following: neglected, abandoned, needy, lonely, desperate, hopeless, helpless, ashamed, guilty, worthless, unlovable, scared, empty, and hollow. They can also give the client a full range of physiological discomfort, such as acute or gnawing pain, shakiness and agitation, intense hunger or lack of appetite. When these parts are retrieved from their exile and cared for, they can feel elated, devoted, adoring, contented, appropriately sad and empathic, and warmly affectionate. Also, they are often highly creative, spontaneous, and playful. In other words, they have the same range of emotions as external children.

Everyone has these child-like parts, so this description of them should be familiar to the reader. In many clients, however (although not unlike many other people), these parts are often burdened by extreme ideas about themselves and are stuck at some extreme point in the client's past. Within the client's internal system, the managers isolate exiles from the Self and from many other parts. Thus, these child-like parts are chronically neglected in the internal system; consequently, they are constantly vulnerable to becoming terribly upset. In addition, many clients have other parts that disdain these inner children and make the clients feel ashamed to have them. So these child-like parts are not only neglected; they are also chronically disapproved of and criticized internally. This only confirms the negative beliefs they have about themselves that come from the past.

Given that such a client has what feels like a reservoir of pain, desperation, shame, and bad memories, it is no wonder that the client's internal system organizes to keep him or her away from these parts. Managers believe that if the door to these feelings is opened, the client will be sucked into a black hole of pain and despair, never to return. Commonly, the client's managers also believe that these feelings are immutable, so the only solution is to keep them dissociated (shut off somewhere), and to avoid activating them by avoiding external stimuli that might trigger their feelings. Other parts sit, like firefighters awaiting an alarm, ready to jump into action if these child-like parts are activated, so as to quickly distract from or anesthetize these parts. The firefighters will do anything to achieve their mission, as described in Chapter 2. For bulimic clients, the method of first choice is usually food. If food doesn't work, however, these parts may resort to other measures—drugs or alcohol, sex, self-cutting, or stealing.

Blending

What the managers and the firefighters fear is flooding of the exiles' feelings, thoughts, or sensations, so that they blend with the person's Self or permeate the entire system. That is, if given an opportunity, parts have the ability to erase the boundary separating them from other parts or the Self. When a part infuses its feelings into the Self, it obscures the Self's resources and, in a sense, merges with the Self or takes control of the system. It is important to remember that this blending of Self and exiles is the main thing the managers and firefighters fear (except in cases where the exiles are carrying secrets and there is the fear that these secrets will be revealed).

Why are managers and firefighters so afraid of the blending? There are several reasons. When the Self blends with the feelings of a child-like exile, the Self becomes overwhelmed with the part's pain, despair, or fear; as a result, the Self stops leading, and the system feels much more vulnerable. In addition, the child-like exiles usually are desperate to find, and will idealize, some external person whom they think can take care of them. Or the exiles may carry the burden of worthlessness and may be looking for redemption from someone resembling the person who originally made them feel worthless. As a result, the blended client repeatedly rushes into relationships and gets rejected or hurt in worse ways.

Finally, child-like exiles are often surrounded by firefighters who react powerfully to any sign that the children are upset. In some cases then, managers are not afraid of the child-like exiles per se, but instead fear the release of firefighters who use rash, destructive methods to "help" the exiles. The most common fear is the release of rage, which, in a person who has been abused, may result in the person's abusing someone else or in being hurt by other people's reactions to the rage. Also, if child parts have a strong need to be redeemed by the abuser, the release of rage will end all hope for redemption, because the recognition of what the abuser did is revealed and the person may leave that relationship.

For people who were chronically abused, managers also fear the release of a part whose job it is to get them to commit suicide. Often one part has been given responsibility for putting a permanent end to the pain if it becomes intolerable or to keep secrets secret. These suicide parts can also be triggered when exiles are exposed. Other feared reactions include typical firefighter activities of self-mutilation, or bingeing on food, drugs, alcohol, sex. Thus, all these firefighters lurk like hidden bombs that can be triggered by opening the door to the exiles prematurely. Rightfully, managers resist the efforts of well-meaning therapists to pry the door open until these bombs have been defused.

In sum, blending of child-like exiles can result in pain and vulnerability—two things that managers and firefighters are organized to keep a person free from. It is important to remember that blending per se is not destructive. In fact, it is important for many exiled parts to have their feelings experienced by the Self at some point. Once these feelings have been experienced, the exiles have the sense that they have been fully accepted. What happened to them is more fully acknowledged and can be less easily denied when the person feels the emotions and sensations than when these are experienced as merely memories or movie-like images.

The timing of the blending is what I am urging caution about here. A premature sharing of the exiles' intense feelings such that the Self is overwhelmed can have several negative consequences. First, if the Self feels as scared, sad, or young as the exile, the Self is no longer able to comfort and reassure it. Second, a manager may quickly shut down the system and punish the person or distance from the therapist. Third, hairtrigger firefighters may explode, leading to dangerous impulsive behaviors. For these reasons, it is best to keep the exiles from overwhelming the Self during initial efforts to help them.

Clients often find another analogy useful in understanding how the Self can experience some of a part's feelings without being overwhelmed:

Body surfers know that they will remain safe, even in large waves, as long as they keep their heads out of the water. The second their head is submerged, however, they are dashed against the sand. Similarly, it is usually safe for the Self to be carried by a part's waves of feeling as long as it is not totally submerged. It is the total immersion that the system fears.

Thus, releasing exiles can be a delicate operation. Yet one major goal of the IFS model is for the Self to ensure that the hurt child-like exiles are cared for. Caring for them often includes the Self's witnessing, listening to, and empathizing with their stories of what happened to them; helping them leave the past and release the burdens they have accumulated, so they can live comfortably in the present; holding their bodies; comforting their fears; accepting their flaws; playing with them; visiting them on a regular basis and whenever they are upset; and setting them up with other parts who can look after them when the Self is busy. In other words, the Self does for them what a caring adult would do for abandoned or traumatized children.

When the Self is able to do this on a consistent basis, these parts return to their nonextreme states; they become normal children again. Thus, contrary to the beliefs of managers, these child-like exiles can change, and often rather quickly. They and their extreme feelings do not have to be walled off once they are taken care of. Indeed, it is the walling off that maintains their extremes. In sum, sharing the exile's feelings is often vital but should not occur until the Self can do so without losing its own boundaries and blending completely with the exiles.

Collaborating with Managers

Given all the valid concerns of the managers over the blending of the child-like exiles, how can the exiles be released and cared for safely? For managers to relax enough to allow the Self access to exiles, they must be convinced that if they open the door to the exiles, the following will happen (or not happen):

assuage manager concerns

1. The Self can help the exiles; these horrible feelings will change.
2. The Self will not be overwhelmed—this can be done without blending with the exiles.
3. Dangerous firefighters will not be triggered.
4. The therapist will not be repulsed by the exiles and will not lose respect for, abandon, or punish the client for exposing them.
5. The client's external environment is safe enough to expose exiles; there are not dangerous parts of people in his or her life that will

react hurtfully to their exposure (and if the client is attacked, the Self will help the exiles).

6. The exposure of any secrets the exiles hold will not result in dire consequences, such as death, reabuse, or the loss of any chance for redemption from or connection to family members.

7. The managers themselves will not be eliminated once they are no longer needed in their overprotective roles.

If the managers can be convinced of these these things, they will give the Self access, and in fact will help rather than resist the therapist.

Not every manager has all of these concerns, but these are the most common ones, and it behooves the therapist to explore them thoroughly. Below, I offer ways to address each of these concerns.

Providing Reassurance That Exiles Can Change

Many managers will insist that there is no point to working with the client's pain, because "the damage has been done and cannot be undone, so all you can do is stay away from the pain and not look back." An embodiment of this managerial philosophy was the late Richard Nixon, who, when asked about the secret to his longevity in a recent interview, stated: "My view is, 'Never look back, always look to the future because if you look to the future you may live to enjoy it. Look back and you die'" (*Chicago Tribune*, Jan. 10, 1993).

To counter this belief, I reassure the managers that although I understand why they believe this, it is not true:

"The parts that hold your pain and fear can change if they are taken care of. Their extreme state is the result of being stuck in the past and of having been exiled. Once retrieved and cared for, they will let go of their extreme feelings and will be valuable, enjoyable parts, and you [the managers] will not have to stay in this extreme role of trying to keep them out."

It may take some time, persistence, and experimenting before managers are willing to consider this possibility.

Controlling Blending

The most important discovery in the IFS model in the past several years is the way to achieve the second of those concerns: how to bring the Self into proximity with a part without totally blending—that is, without overwhelming the Self with the part's feelings. The answer to this problem is quite simple, but as is true of so many things, the simple answers are often the hardest to see. It turns out that parts can control the release of their feelings, and can thus maintain their boundaries, if they believe that it is in their best interest to do so. Thus, the Self can get close to a child-like part without being overwhelmed by its feelings if the part decides not to blend with the Self—that is, decides to contain its feelings within itself to some degree. The overwhelming will not occur if the part sees a good reason not to blend totally.

Why do hurt parts want to blend? They usually report several reasons, all of them quite valid. First, they want the feelings out of themselves. Second, they want the Self to know how they feel and what they have been through; like members of any oppressed group, they want to break through their walls and be liberated and accepted. Third, they hope that in taking over, they can make the client find an external person who will take care of or redeem them. Fourth, they are afraid that they will be exiled again by managerial parts as soon as they give up the control they have gained from the blending.

This fourth reason illustrates the vicious cycle between managerial and child-like exiles that perpetuates their isolation. The more they try to blend, the more the managers try to keep them exiled, the more they try to blend, and so on. For some clients this cycle results in a constant alternation of control between the managerial and the hurt child-like parts, so that the clients appear emotionally labile—crying and needy one moment, and coldly detached or hostile the next. It is as if they alternate between two entirely different and separate worlds: one barren and grim, the other desperately lonely, painful, and chaotic. For other clients, one or the other group predominates for an extended period, until the disenfranchised group is activated enough to throw a coup.

The therapist or the client's Self must try to explain to the client's child-like parts that although their attempts to blend totally are understandable, such attempts are not in their best interest. If they blend, the Self will feel as upset and impotent as they do and will not be able to help them, and the managerial parts will exile them again. If they keep their feelings and thoughts somewhat separated, the Self can help them and the managers will not fear them. Frequently, these hurt parts can understand the reasons pertaining to the managers, but have trouble believing or trusting that the Self can help them. This is because the Self has not been able to help these young ones in the past, which is why they have looked to other people. Often, however, they can be convinced to give this at least a try.

With such an agreement in place, the therapist asks the client's Self first to ask the managers not to interfere, and then to approach a child-like part but stop where the Self begins to feel overwhelmed by the part's feelings. Sometimes the child part is cooperating to such an extent that the Self can get very close and even hold the part immediately. More often, the Self has to stop several times and remind the part not to overwhelm it before they can become close. Sometimes this takes more than one session.

Throughout this process, the managers should be consulted as to how they think things are going. They also should be encouraged to let the therapist or the client's Self know if they become highly concerned. If managers are shown this kind of respect, they can become cooperative consultants who give advice and monitor the pace. Thus, the IFS model views what has been traditionally called "resistance" as the managerial parts' often valid fears about people entering their delicate system. They do not resist, and can help, if they are respected and are convinced that the therapist knows how to work safely.

Addressing the Fear of Releasing Dangerous Firefighters

As described earlier, working with hurt, child-like exiles can trigger the release of rageful, suicidal, or otherwise impulsive firefighters. Frequently the managers' resistance to letting the Self work with these vulnerable child parts stems not so much from fear of their blending as from fear that the firefighters may be triggered by the process. Frequently, also, managers do not bring up these fears because they prefer to pretend that the firefighters do not exist. The therapist will be wise, then, to ask the managers specifically about fears of rage, suicide, bingeing, or the like. Even when managers deny such fears, the therapist should remain vigilant for evidence of firefighters. In cases where they exist and are inhibiting the work, the therapist will need to work with them first to defuse their scary, destructive potential. More details on how to work with firefighters are provided in Chapter 5.

Trust in the Therapist

Many clients have a history in which, whenever they trusted other people enough to expose their exiles, they were hurt or abandoned by those people (previous therapists included). Thus, they have good reason to fear that the same will be true of their present therapist. The client's managers (or their exiles themselves) may have adopted the attitude of significant others that the exiles are extremely repulsive, disgusting, or overwhelming. Thus they are convinced that exposure of these exiles will certainly kill their relationship with the therapist.

Unfortunately, with many therapists, these fears of abandonment or scorn are well founded. Many therapists have trouble with their own exiles, and consequently react to their clients' exiles with their own managers. When such therapists' protective managers take over, it is extremely distressing for many clients, especially if they have exposed or are about to expose exiles. It is as if the safe, caring, and warm people they thought they were opening up to have suddenly been transformed into cold, hostile, or unfeeling people, often confirming their sense of worthlessness and hopelessness. When this happens, clients are likely to respond with their own protective managers or with their increasingly desperate exiles, triggering an escalation with the therapists' parts.

This speaks to the importance of therapists' doing enough work with their own parts that they can maintain Self-leadership with all their clients' parts. Therapists should not work with exiles until this is true, and until they can sincerely assure their clients that they will not be rejected, abandoned, or punished. In my case, once the gates are opened and exiles are exposed, I feel a tremendous responsibility to the client. I will not open the door until I am sure I can maintain this commitment to be there no matter what.

The distrusting managers of many clients are not calmed by one or two reassurances. Instead, concerns over trust arise continually, particularly as the therapist is gradually allowed to come closer. Many clients want to be assured that the therapist really cares about them, beyond just doing a job. Many therapists are trained to deflect these requests and to remain opaque regarding their feelings. Such opaqueness only heightens the clients' distrust and prolongs the process. Instead, I find ways to reassure clients that I do care about them, including telling them so. The IFS model helps in this regard, because even when people are led by obnoxious parts, I know that they have (and I can usually access) other, more likable parts or their Selves. Thus, it is rare that I cannot tell a client sincerely that I care about him or her; in a case where I do not feel that way, I can say that this is because we have not yet really met.

The opaque position is based on the fear that a therapist's direct expressions of caring promote unrealistic or inappropriate fantasies in clients or take away the pressure to explore the need to be cared for. The IFS model helps with these concerns as well, because both therapist and client know that only the young parts of the client need the reassurance and may have fantasies. Also, the client has a Self who can help these young parts with their needs and fantasies, and who, with the therapist, can encourage these parts to show where they are frozen in time—how they became so scared and needy. Thus, I can reassure a client that I care about him or her, and can also ask the client to find the parts that are so worried about that. Then I can help those parts see that they can also look to the client's Self for that reassurance.

Addressing External Concerns

It is unwise, if not unethical, to bring exiles back into a dangerous environment. If a client lives with an abusive spouse or other family member, I will try to change that environment before or while working with the client's parts. If managers are resisting IFS therapy, it may be that they will not let the therapist in until they have a safe world in which to bring back hurt parts. Even if the client's spouse or family members are not particularly abusive, they may respond in extreme ways as the client does the work and as various parts emerge or exert more influence, or as the client becomes stronger and less dependent. For these reasons, it is crucial that the therapist and client thoroughly assess—and, if necessary and possible, change—the client's external context before and during this internal work. I frequently wind up working with the parts of external family members that are activated by the client's parts. Chapter 7 is largely devoted to assessing and changing external contexts.

Dealing with the Fear of Exposing Secrets

Sometimes exiled parts not only hold difficult feelings, but also hold secrets about a person's life that are unacceptable or threaten the person or the external family. The revelation of these secrets may indeed produce major changes in relationships, so managers have good reason to fear them. Many times, however, fear of the secrets is anachronistic. It is the product of threats made to the person as a child, or of fears that family members conveyed that are no longer relevant. Without asking for the secrets to be revealed, the therapist can explore with the client's managers what they fear would happen if the secrets were revealed. Together, the therapist's and client's Selves and the client's managers can assess the current validity of those fears and plan ways to address them if they are currently valid.

Some managers fear that if they face how the client was hurt in the past by a significant person, they would have to believe that this person never loved the client, and the client would be left with chronic feelings of unlovability. Or they would have to confront, cut off from, or betray a person on whom the client still depends. The IFS model helps address both of these concerns. First, the client learns that everyone, abusers included, has different parts. Some parts of the client's abuser were once hurt and later wanted to hurt others. Other parts, however, may have loved the client a great deal. The fact that the other person was abusive does not negate the love.

Second, through the IFS model, the client can heal without actually confronting the person who hurt him or her. This assertion is contrary to a popular and pernicious myth in the sexual abuse field—namely, the belief that in order for a survivor of sexual abuse to heal completely, the abuser must acknowledge and apologize for the abuse. With this belief, the survivor remains dependent on the actions of the abuser. In addition, too many clients are encouraged to confront their abusers prematurely— well before their internal systems are ready to handle the abusers' reactions or before the validity of the abuse memories is clear. As a result, they are reabused emotionally by denial or counterattack.

People feel empowered to learn that they are no longer dependent on the actions of others to heal. They are also glad to learn that (except in cases where abuse is still going on) they have a great deal of control over decisions regarding whether, when, and how to confront. If a decision to confront is made, a therapist and client should spend as much time as needed preparing the client internally, so that the client's Self remains in the lead and parts are not hurt no matter how the interaction goes.

Addressing the Fear That Managers Will Be Eliminated

Many parts believe that they *are* their roles. That is, they have been in extreme roles for so long and have been so preoccupied with them that they are unaware of any other feelings, desires, or talents they possess. As a result, they are convinced that once the need for their roles is gone, *they* will be gone. Also, sometimes their roles have been so oppressive and destructive that other parts are eager to eliminate them and may jump at the chance to do so. The therapist or the client's Self can help managers discover that they are much more than their roles by asking about what they would like to do once the need for their protectiveness is reduced. They can be reassured that new, valued roles are available once they feel safe enough to change.

In summary, the main point of this section is that managers often have legitimate fears and should be treated with respect. The IFS model has developed ways to address each of these common fears, and managers should be given as much attention as necessary to allay their fears. Because some managers seem so manipulative, destructive, or belligerent, they can easily activate protective or controlling parts of the therapist. When this happens, an escalation will be triggered between the therapist's and the client's managers that at best will impede progress, and at worst can be dangerous. If the client's protective managers are not respected, or their concerns at least considered, they will sabotage the therapy and may punish the client. The danger lies in this punishment; depending on the vulnerability of the system being protected, it can range from internal criticism to dangerous physiological reactions or self-destructive acts. As a result of witnessing some of these dangerous reactions, I have learned to be respectful of protective managers.

There are other managers who appear to be very reasonable and helpful. They often convey much knowledge about the inner system and encourage the therapist to rely on them. They seem so rational that they can be confused with the person's Self. It is tempting to overpromote these parts and put them in charge of others, but this is a mistake. Despite their helpful demeanor, they may have their own agenda, which is often to keep certain exiles buried by leading therapy away from them.

Retrieving Parts That Are "Frozen in Time"

Once the managers are reassured to some degree about these and any other fears, and have agreed to give some access to exiles, the therapist asks the person's Self to find an exile. That is, the Self may just ask for an exiled part to appear inside; alternately, it may have to focus on an exiled feeling (often fear, sadness, anger, grief, loneliness, or emptiness) or on a body sensation. As the exile emerges (either as an image or as a feeling), the therapist must be careful to prevent it from overwhelming the Self, which might trigger managers to shut down the work. The therapist has the Self ask the exile not to overwhelm the Self as the Self approaches the part. When the exile agrees not to blend, the Self gets as close as possible to it without being overwhelmed by its feelings.

When the Self gets close to a hurt child-like part, often the Self needs to convince this part that the Self cares about it and can be trusted. The Self may also need to spend some time comforting and holding the part during this initial encounter before the part is calm enough to interact. If the Self can demonstrate this caring and consistency, the part will gradually open up and talk about its feelings. Sometimes this kind of attention from the Self or other parts is all the child-like part needs to shift from its extreme state. Most often, however, exiled child parts are stuck somewhere in the past, and so will revert to their extreme state until they can leave that time and place.

Parts who are stuck in the past seem to be stuck at a point in the client's life that was emotion-packed. Child-like parts are often stuck during a period when the person was scared, rejected, humiliated, abandoned, or traumatized, or experienced a loss. The part feels as if it literally lives in that time period, which accounts for the fact that no matter how much attention it receives from the client's Self or from external people, it remains extreme. Only after such a part is retrieved from the past and can be nurtured in the present can it let go of its extreme feelings or beliefs.

To find where an exiled part is frozen in time, the Self simply asks. Before this is done, however, it is important for the Self to be well differentiated and for managers and firefighters not to interfere. The therapist will be wise to ask the client's Self whether the Self is ready to see where the part is stuck and whether other parts are afraid, and then deal with the fears before proceeding.

When asked, most child-like parts can indicate in some way where they are stuck. Some will show a scene to the Self; others will verbally describe their surroundings; still others will give the Self a feeling that is identifiable with a particular time or place. Once the stuck point is located, the person's Self asks the part to show or say everything it wants to about what happened. Once the part is finished telling or showing its story, the therapist asks the Self to enter the scene and be with the part in the way that the client wished someone had been there when it really happened. The part is asked what burdens it accumulated from this experience and whether it would like to leave those burdens there (see the section on unburdening, below). Then the exile is asked whether it is ready to leave that place and time and come into the present with the Self, or whether it needs to do or say anything to anyone there first. The exile is also asked whether there is anything it wants to leave there or bring with it.

If the part does not want to leave, this usually means that (1) it does not yet trust that the Self can care for it; (2) there are people or parts in the client's present life that seem dangerous to it; or (3) there is something (a person or a feeling) about that point in the past that the part is not ready to leave. If the Self can visit the part consistently in the past or make the present safer, then the part will gradually want to leave the stuck point. If the part has things to resolve about that point in the past, it can live in the present but visit the past with the Self until it understands what happened and is ready to let go of this. I usually try to bring a stuck part into the present as soon as it is willing to go, rather than leaving it in the past until everything there is resolved. If a traumatized part can rest and heal in the present, then it will have an easier time understanding what happened to it and bringing that perspective with it on any return visits.

It is worth noting that as a result of this retrieval work, I am much more respectful of how past events or interactions impact clients than I was as a structural/strategic family therapist. Part of my previous reluctance to do in-depth explorations of people's pasts in search of insights was the imprecise and lengthy nature of such expeditions. This retrieval work with parts remedies those concerns. It is extremely precise and quick, and I do not have to do any of the searching or interpreting myself.

In other words, the parts generally know what happened to make them so extreme, and if the stage is set properly, they will tell or show the person's Self and the therapist.

Sometimes when a child-like part is asked where it is stuck, the managers react violently and immediately to the question. This often indicates that there are secrets about what happened at that past time that the protective parts are hiding. These secrets often involve abuse, and they are hidden not only from external people but also from the client's Self. Protective parts have a variety of reasons for hiding secrets. Often they are afraid that the Self will not be able to handle the information—that the self will blend with rageful, sad, or suicidal parts activated by the memories. Sometimes they are protecting the identity of the abuser. They may have been given that burden by the abuser, who told the client as a child that terrible things would happen if his or her identity were revealed. Sometimes the managers are certain that the abuse made the client evil, damaged, or repulsive, and he or she will be abandoned by anyone who discovers his or her true nature. They have been given the burden of shame.

In the preceding section, I have presented a variety of ways to address managers' fears about releasing secrets. I might add that managers are like internal censors; they have some control over the way information is released within the inner system, especially if the exile that holds the memories or sensations is willing to cooperate. The memories can be released in flashbacks or in dreams; the content can be an actual reliving of the experience or a metaphoric representation of it; the managers and the exile can release just the images without the feelings or sensations, or just the sensations without any images or feelings; they can control the clarity of the images and the pace at which each memory is released. All of this can be overtly negotiated with whichever managers have most control over this area, so that the memory release is carried out in a safe way and at a safe pace. Just knowing that they will have some control over the pace will help the managers relax.

Throughout this process, it is important that the therapist never voice a guess or suggestion about where the part is stuck or what the secret may be. Some clients have approval-oriented parts that can generate images they think the therapist wants to see, and can produce what have been called "false memories." If the therapist suspects this to be the case, he or she should ask the client to check and see whether such a part is involved, and, if so, why the part feels the need to do this.

Once all this is in place—managers have been consulted and are cooperative, the exile wants to come into the present, the present is a safe place for it to live, and the Self is differentiated enough to care for it—then the part and the Self should discuss the pros and cons of various locations for the part to live. The range of locations is wide. Some parts want, at least for a while, to stay close to the Self and so accompany the person around all day. Other parts are fine if they can stay in the person's bedroom or living room. Others want to live in another house or in another state or country. Some want to stay outside in a pleasant setting or live on an island. It doesn't seem to matter, as long as the part feels safe and can be visited easily by the Self. In addition, if the present does not feel safe, the part can be taken to a different location in the past where the person was safe.

Once a location has been agreed upon, the Self takes the part to the new place, stays with the part there until it feels safe, and tries to arrange things so that the part is comfortable. The Self also asks the part whether it would like for other parts to stay with it there to keep an eye on it when the Self is not there. If the part wants this, then the Self asks for volunteers among the other parts. Frequently, one of the managers volunteers; directly guarding and caretaking then become the part's new role.

The Self then asks the managers how they feel about this change and whether any parts are likely to sabotage it. This includes any parts that might keep the Self from following through and visiting the child part. If the Self doesn't follow through, the consequences can be negative. The child part will feel abandoned and may return to the past, becoming more reluctant than ever to leave; moreover, the managers will lose trust in the Self. It is important, therefore, to make sure that the Self will be able to follow through, and this applies to any agreements made with child parts.

Despite all precautions, there will be times when a part goes, or is thrust, back to the place where it was stuck. When this happens, the therapist and the client's Self need to explore with the exile and managers why this happened and what needs to change so that the exile can stay after it is retrieved again.

As a final note, I have focused here on the retrieval of exiled hurt parts, but it is important to remember that for some clients many if not all parts (including managers and firefighters) are frozen in the past and need retrieving at some point.

Unburdening

As described in Chapter 2, parts of people accumulate burdens as they go through their lives. These burdens take the form of extreme ideas or feelings that govern the parts' existence. Because these burdens are not intrinsic to the parts and instead are placed on or in them, they can be unloaded.

Some clients object to the whole concept of burdens. They see unburdening as too gimmicky, too easy. They do not want to believe that things they have struggled with all their lives can just be lifted out of them. If this were possible, they would blame themselves for carrying the burdens so long and not taking them out earlier. Or they may strongly adhere to the belief that burdens are irreversibly intertwined in their being. Others may fear that once a part is unburdened, the therapist will assume that this is all the part needs and will neglect it. Some abuse survivors react severely to the suggestion that anything was put into them. Their young parts misunderstand the concept of burdens and assume it means they have been violated by something physical. For these reasons, therapists need to be sensitive in the way they describe and approach unburdening. They should assure clients that there was no way for them to have released the burdens on their own, and that (as we shall see) it is not always so easy to do so. But it is also crucial for therapists to maintain the conviction that burdens are not intrinsic to parts and can eventually be jettisoned. Therapists can say with all sincerity, "There is nothing bad inside of you that is *you*. You were born good, and anything in there that seems shameful or destructive was pumped into you by people or events. We can pump it back out."

For unburdening to occur, then, a part needs to recognize that the burden is not the part's essence, but instead came from the outside. This realization happens most often during the retrieval process described above, because as the scene in which a part is stuck is recounted or replayed, the way the burden was imposed on the part becomes clearer to all involved. For some parts, however, this realization takes more time and discussion with the therapist. They can only believe it when they have come to trust the therapist in general.

Once the part can recognize that it is carrying a burden, the Self asks the part to find where the burden is located in or on the part: "Where on or in your body do you carry this feeling or thought?" Most parts can quickly find the burden and are happy to take it off. The Self asks the part to take off the burden and do with it whatever feels correct. There is great variation in what a part takes off and what is done with this. For example, one client's part, carrying the burden of worthlessness, took off some dirty clothes and buried them in the woods. Another client's part found a sticky, dark paste covering the top of her heart, scooped it off, and gave it back to the man who had abused her. Often parts carry several different burdens or received the same burden from several sources, so they may need to repeat this process. It is remarkable, however, how quickly parts can be liberated once they find and remove their burdens.

In some cases, the part unloads and disposes of its burdens, feels much better, and lives happily ever after. Sometimes, however, there are snags. The part itself may be afraid to unload the burden, or other parts may be invested in keeping it. For example, parts may fear that if the burden of worthlessness is gone, a part carrying the burden of rage may be released. The worthlessness has been containing the rage and turning it inward toward safer targets. Before the worthlessness can be released, the rage has to be unburdened.

Thus, it is not uncommon to find that after an apparently successful unburdening, the burden has returned. When that is the case, the client's Self simply asks what happened and why (i.e., discovers the piece of the inner ecology not dealt with initially), and then addresses the fears of the parts that have put the burden back. Like anything else in internal systems, burdens can become deeply embedded in the ecology and can serve seemingly critical functions.

Once exiles have been retrieved from the past and have shed their burdens, it is time for them to be reunited with the rest of the internal family. It is important for the managers and firefighters to see that these exiles have changed and no longer have to be feared or protected. It is also important that new relationships among all parts be forged as each leaves its old, extreme role and finds a new, preferred role that fits with the larger group. As this happens, there are no longer managers, exiles, and firefighters; there are just internal family members.

Summary

To summarize this chapter, I present a list of the common factors that constrain any part from adopting its preferred role and keep it in an extreme role. When I meet a part for the first time, most of my questions revolve around this list as I explore with the part why it does what it does.

1. The part is polarized with one or more other parts. It fears that if it decreases its extremeness, it will be overtaken or eliminated, or will lose its position. For example, an anxious manager may refuse to stop giving panic attacks, for fear that the person's rageful exile may take over.

2. The part is protecting one or more other parts. If it changes, it fears some other part will be harmed. The same anxious manager may also fear that if it cuts back on the panic attacks, the person will have the courage to ask someone out on a date and be rejected, which will hurt some exiles.

3. The part is stuck in the past. For example, the anxious part lives during a time when the person was a young child whose father and mother had scary fights.

4. The part carries burdens. For example, the part inherited the burden of worry from the person's mother, who was constantly afraid that her husband might explode.

5. There is something in the person's external environment that is activating the part. For example, the person works in an office where everyone lives with the constant threat of losing his or her job. In addition, the person's spouse denies this threat and continues to spend carelessly.

6. There is something in the relationship between the therapist and client that is activating the part. For example, the therapist never directly communicates his or her caring, so the person's anxious part constantly worries about the therapist's disapproval.

Some parts are confined to their extreme roles by only one or two of these factors; many others, however, are constrained by all of them. When I meet a part, then, I often ask about many of these possible constraints. Then, with the person's Self, I begin to try to change them, one by one, until the part is able to remain in its preferred role. In the case of the anxious part described above, I may first try to depolarize its relationship with the angry part, then to retrieve the exiles it protects, and then to retrieve and unburden the anxious part itself, all the while addressing issues in our relationship or in the external environment that may be activating it.

The point is that one intervention is rarely enough by itself to release a part from its extreme role. The therapist often needs persistence and patience. This list of constraining factors can help guide that persistence.

CHAPTER 5

Methods of Inner Work: In-Sight and Direct Access

There are numerous ways to access and work with a person's internal system. The IFS model emphasizes two: "in-sight" and "direct access." I am aware, however, that many other methods exist. Some methods are more esoteric, including forms of massage or shamanic ritual; others are more traditional, including various projective techniques such as the sand tray or psychodrama. No doubt there are many ways waiting to be discovered.

We are always limited by our methods. The methods I emphasize in this chapter are those with which I have worked the most extensively and am most comfortable. They work well for me and for many of the people I have trained, but undoubtedly contain constraints that could be released by other methods. Therefore, by emphasizing these methods, I do not want to limit other possibilities by discouraging readers from trying alternatives; it is just that I cannot speak as clearly about the safe application of alternatives. I urge that the reader proceed carefully, keeping in mind some of the general cautions included in Chapter 4, as well as those described at the end of this chapter.

In-sight

Frequently, much of what is described in Chapter 3 is carried out through what might be called "imagery." Imagery is not the best term for this work, however, because the client usually is not trying to or being told to imagine anything; as is the case in various forms of guided imagery. Instead, it is as if through focusing internally, the client is entering and seeing a world that already exists. I use the term "in-sight" to describe this process, because of its literal denotation of "inner vision" and because of its more common connotation of "keen understanding," which is what the method can produce.

I stumbled into this method of working with internal systems after my clients began telling me that they could see their parts and could see them interacting. I later learned that Jung (see Hannah, 1981) had experimented with a similar process, which he called "active imagination"; this process has been refined by Robert Johnson (1986).

At this point in the IFS model's development, much of the internal work with clients is done through in-sight, because I have found it to be an extremely efficient modality. Through in-sight, a client can often quickly identify a large number of parts and can quickly differentiate the Self. The client can also do "internal family therapy"—that is, work with his or her parts as a group, with the Self acting as therapist to the family of parts. In addition, clients can engage in in-sight between sessions on their own, which heightens their ability to change themselves and lessens their dependence on the therapist.

Initially, some clients are better than others at seeing this inner world clearly. Some immediately see their parts with amazing clarity; for others, the parts are quite fuzzy; and a minority of clients cannot see anything. I have found that the initial difficulty clients have is often traceable to the influence of certain parts that inhibit this in-sight. For example, people who are dominated by highly rational, analytic, striving parts; by parts that worry a great deal about whether they are performing well; or by parts that do not trust the therapist or the process often have difficulty at first. If, however, such people are able to calm and separate from the inhibiting parts so that they no longer interfere, it is not uncommon for them to find that suddenly they are able to see internally. ("Seeing" is not always the proper term for this process, because while for some clients it is like watching a Technicolor movie, for others it is less a vision than a kind of sense that these things are happening.)

Clients who never really see their parts can sense their presence and can interact with them without visualizing them. It is not crucial for a client to see his or her parts to do in-sight work. All that is required is that the client have a sense of where the part is.

Getting Started

The first step in helping a client enter this world is to ask him or her to focus on a part. Before a client and I get to that step, however, usually we have been using the parts language for some time, and the client has indicated a wish to change his or her relationship with certain parts. I have said that there are many ways to do this, one of which is through imagery (I use the term "imagery," rather than "in-sight," with clients because they are generally more comfortable with it), and the client has agreed to try it. I ask which part the client wants to begin with, and he or she selects one. If the part selected is likely to be a manager, we proceed. If it is likely to be an exile or firefighter, I ask the client to find parts that might be afraid for us to work with the exile or firefighter, and we work with these parts first.

THERAPIST: What part would you like to start with?

MARY: I guess the part that's so critical of me.

THERAPIST: Okay, focus on that part of you, however you experience it. If it is a feeling, focus on the feeling. If it's a thought pattern or an inner voice, focus on that. If it seems to be a sensation located in a place in your body, focus on that place. As you focus on this part, see if an image for it comes to you. Don't try images on—just wait for the part to show itself to you. If you hear a voice saying you're no good at imagery or that this is stupid, or that I don't know what I'm doing, or anything else that seems to be interfering, ask the part that is saying that to trust you for a little while and not interfere. If you are not getting an image, that's okay, because we can do this without your seeing the part.

MARY: I'm not sure that this is what you want, but I see an old woman—it looks like a witch and she's scowling at me.

In this case, the client saw a part immediately. Other clients are unable to see a part. There are many reasons for this: The part may be afraid to be seen, or may be too highly identified with or close to the Self to be seen; other parts are still inhibiting the process; or a client can sense but not see the parts. In the last-mentioned case, a client can often still work with the part, even though it is invisible. The client can ask the part why it won't show itself, or ask other parts why they won't let it appear, and try to deal with the answers. More often, however, the work simply proceeds as though the clients can see the part. For example, in doing the "room technique" (to be described more fully below), the therapist simply asks the client to move the part into a room by itself, even though he or she cannot see it. Thus, the client moves the feeling, voice, thought, or sensation into a room and is asked to be outside the room. Once the part is separated from the Self in this way, it is easier for the Self to work with it, and the client is frequently able to see it shortly after putting it into the room.

The Room Technique

I learned the hard way that in many cases, it is important to separate the original part from the Self and other parts immediately, so that the Self can form a personal relationship with it before dealing with its polarized relationship to other parts. Before learning to do this, I found that for some clients, the part they saw would suddenly attack them or quickly run away and hide. The simplest way to prevent these reactions and achieve this separation is to have a client, soon after he or she sees the part, put it in a room by itself and look at it from outside the room through a window.

Occasionally, a part will react strongly against being put into a room. This may occur for many reasons; in one example, the person's mother used to put her in a closet as a child. The room is not essential. All that is important is to achieve some kind of initial separation; thus, the part can go out into a field or some other place that feels comfortable to it. In addition, it is not always necessary to begin in-sight with the room technique. When a client has a less polarized and more differentiated internal system, I skip this step and just have the client begin working with his or her parts without any separation.

THERAPIST: Okay, Mary, now put the Witch in a room by itself, and you stay outside the room.

MARY: Okay, she's in there.

Just this act of separating from a part can be very significant for a client. From this vantage point outside the room, the person can, often for the first time, consider the part without blending with its feelings and can see that it is different from the Self. The next step in this technique is to further differentiate the client's Self from other parts, particularly those parts that are polarized with the part in the room—in Mary's case, the Witch. If these polarized parts do not separate from the Self, then it is very difficult to get anything to change between the original part and the Self.

The principle here is the same as in the structural family therapy technique of boundary making (Minuchin & Fishman, 1981). As noted earlier, when one wants to improve the relationship between two external family members, one tries to improve the boundary around their relationship by getting other family members not to interfere when the original dyad interacts. For example, a father is asked to keep quiet while his wife and daughter talk about how they can get along better.

Using this boundary-making principle internally, I found that if I had the client find and separate from a part who was polarized with the original part, the person's perception of and feelings toward the original part would change immediately and dramatically. After experimenting with this technique for some time, I discovered that if I moved enough parts, the client would invariably reach a state of mind in which he or she felt either compassion, curiosity, or acceptance regarding the part in the room. This was one of the major discoveries of the IFS model—that this compassionate, confident core, which I call the Self, exists and can be quickly differentiated in this way. I credit my background in family therapy for permitting this discovery.

To begin this differentiation process, the therapist asks the client how he or she feels toward the part in the room as the client looks at it from outside the room. If the client responds with any feeling other than something approaching compassion, acceptance, or curiosity, then it is likely that polarized parts are influencing the Self's view of the original part. The therapist simply asks the client to find the part or parts making him or her feel that way, and to ask them respectfully to separate from the Self so that they will stop influencing him or her.

THERAPIST: How do you feel toward this Witch?

MARY: I'm afraid of her. She can make me feel terrible.

THERAPIST: Find the part that's afraid of her and ask it to trust you for a few minutes and not to interfere. If you need to, you can move it into another room and ask it to wait until you're done.

MARY: (*After a pause*) Okay.

THERAPIST: How do you feel toward the Witch now?

MARY: I'm very angry with it. I wish I could get rid of it—it dominates my life so much.

THERAPIST: Okay, find that angry part and ask it to move also so it doesn't interfere. . . . Good. Now do you feel toward the Witch?

MARY: She has changed. She just looks like a tired old lady. I feel sorry for her.

Before Mary's Self could see the Witch in perspective, she had to move two parts that were polarized with it. Sometimes clients have to move as many as six or seven parts before they are differentiated enough to work effectively with the first part. The key indication of differentiation is the person's response to the question "How do you feel toward the part?" If the client's Self is separate from the influence of interfering parts, the answer will reflect qualities of the Self, both in content and in tone of voice. It is not essential for the Self to be totally differentiated—that is, separated from all other parts. It just needs to be differentiated enough to have a positive or at least open attitude about the part in the room.

Once the client reports feeling compassion or curiosity for the target part, the therapist asks the client to enter the room, approach the part, and interact with it about his or her relationship with it. If during this process the person sees himself or herself enter the room, then he or she is watching a part do the work rather than the Self. That is, in in-sight, the Self is invisible in the sense that the client should be able to see his or her parts but not himself or herself, just as I can see the computer I am writing this on or the people in the other room, but I cannot see myself. If the client is watching himself or herself interact with the parts, the therapist should ask the client to be there instead and tell the part that is doing the work to trust the Self.

Once the Self is in the room, the therapist should continue to monitor the way the Self is feeling, to be sure that polarized parts have not followed the Self into the room or that the Self is not blending with the target part (see the discussion of blending in Chapter 4). If the Self reports any extreme feelings, or if the target part seems extremely afraid of or agitated by the presence of the Self, the therapist should find any interfering parts and have them leave the room. If the Self is feeling the target part's feelings to a troublesome extent, the Self can ask the part to stop blending. If it does not comply, the Self may have to leave until the part agrees not to overwhelm. In other words, doing this work safely and effectively depends on the Self's being differentiated enough that things go smoothly. When this is not the case, it is worth the extra time to stop and find interfering parts.

This highlights a key assumption: Any time there is trouble in this work, parts are interfering, although it may not be clear immediately whose parts they are (they may be the therapist's). Common problems that novice IFS therapists do not recognize as parts' interference include a client's suddenly losing the image or becoming otherwise distracted, becoming impatient with the pace or with the therapist, or feeling as though a part is correct in its extreme position. In such a case, the therapist simply asks the client to find the part that is creating the interference, and the therapist also looks inside himself or herself to find interference. When I find that one of my own parts is the problem, I relate this to the client. It seems to be helpful to my clients to know that I, too, am actively involved in this work, and to have their perception that I was not my Self confirmed.

Sometimes when the client asks an interfering part to leave, it refuses. This indicates that the intensity of the polarization is strong and that the refusing part does not fully trust the Self's leadership. In such cases, the focus may have to shift temporarily to the refusing part, as the Self asks the part why it is so afraid to leave and works with it around that issue.

After the Self has entered the room and is able to interact with the target part to some extent, the Self can ask the part a series of questions that my colleagues and I have found helpful. These questions revolve around discovering the factors constraining the part in its extreme role (see the list of factors at the end of Chapter 4), and exploring what kind of role it would prefer. With critical, judgmental, striving, or perfectionistic managers, or with indulgent firefighters, questions include the following:

- Why are you doing or saying _____ [the extreme behavior or thought]?
- What is it that you really want for [person's name]?
- What are you afraid would happen if you stopped doing or saying _____?
- If [person's name] were able to keep _____ [the feared consequence named by the part] from happening, so you could do anything you wanted to in the system, what would you want to do?
- Would you like for us to help get you into that new role?

THERAPIST: Go into the room with the Old Lady [formerly the Witch] and ask her why she is so critical of you.

MARY: She says that it's because I make so many mistakes.

THERAPIST: Ask her why she is so concerned with not having you make mistakes.

MARY: She says it's because when I make mistakes, people don't like me. They only like me if I'm perfect.

THERAPIST: Why is it so important to her to have people like you?

MARY: Because if they don't like you, they make fun of you or reject you.

THERAPIST: So ask her what it is that she really wants for you.

MARY: She doesn't want for me to be hurt by people.

THERAPIST: If you could show her that you could take care of the parts that are so hurt when someone rejects or makes fun of you, so they wouldn't be so hurt and vulnerable, would she be interested in finding another role?

MARY: She said that she doesn't believe that I could do that, so it's silly to think about her changing.

THERAPIST: Just suppose for a second that you could, so that the Old Lady wouldn't have to stay in this extreme role and could do anything she wanted. What would she like to do in there?

MARY: She says she would like to take a vacation for a while and just rest.

THERAPIST: Tell her we'll try to help her get a rest.

The reader may have noticed that in this exchange the therapist was quite directive and fed Mary questions to ask the Old Lady. The degree to which the therapist will need to employ this directive stance will vary, but it should be maintained for as brief a time as possible. With many clients, I can shift to a less directive stance soon after the process has begun. To do this, instead of telling a client what to do or say, I ask questions such as "How do you respond to what the part just said?" or "What needs to happen now?" In many cases I have been amazed at how a client's Self, once differentiated, just seems to know how to deal effectively with the whole system and begins telling me what he or she (the Self) is doing rather than asking me what to do. The therapist can test whether the client's Self is ready to take over by occasionally asking nondirective questions and seeing how he or she responds.

When the Self interacts with a hurt child-like exile, the interaction is somewhat different from that with critical, protective, or indulgent managers or with firefighters. With the latter parts, the goal is to help them find their valuable roles and deal with whatever is keeping them from taking these roles. The first objective with child-like parts, in contrast, is usually to take care of them so that they are not so scared or sad.

THERAPIST: (*to Mary's Self*) Can you find the part that the Old Lady is protecting from being rejected or laughed at—the part that feels so hurt when that happens?

MARY: Yeah, it looks like me as a little girl.

THERAPIST: [checking for Self-differentiation] How do you feel toward her?

MARY: She looks so lonely. I wish I could cheer her up.

THERAPIST: [sensing that the Self is differentiated enough] Why don't you try to? See how close you can get to her without being overwhelmed by her.

MARY: (*after a long pause*) She was kind of afraid of me at first and wouldn't tell me how I could help her, but I just sat near her and told her that I would try to take care of her, and finally she crawled up into my lap.

At this point, Mary's Self had clearly taken the lead and knew what to do. It should also be noted that the approach to the child part, the Little Girl, flowed from the work with the Old Lady. The Old Lady was protecting the Little Girl by trying to make Mary perfect so that Mary wouldn't be rejected; in this way, the Little Girl would not be activated.

The IFS model emphasizes the importance of focusing on the networks of relationships among parts, because parts are almost never able to change in isolation. In Mary's case, the Old Lady could not become less extreme until she knew that the Little Girl was no longer so vulnerable and in need of indirect protection. In turn, it would be very difficult for Mary's Self to help the Little Girl as long as the Old Lady was in her critical Witch role, in which she made the Little Girl feel bad and kept the Self away from her. Internal family systems are full of such complementary relationships, which often involve more than just two parts.

As described earlier, it is often the case that parts are frozen in the past or carry burdens, which account for the tenacity of their extreme feelings or beliefs. The reader can refer to the discussions of retrieval and unburdening in Chapter 4 for guidelines regarding these techniques. Through in-sight, unburdening and retrieval can be done efficiently and often with amazing drama.

Internal Family Therapy

So far, I have described using in-sight to change a single part's role or change its relationship with the Self. Some of the most important work with the IFS model, however, involves changing the relationships among the parts. Every client with whom I have worked has parts that are polarized with one another in ways that maintain each part's extremes. One way to address these polarizations is to get the polarized parts to communicate directly. Again, this parallels the structural family therapy techniques of enactment and boundary making, which involve getting two polarized family members to face and talk to each other while the therapist ensures that they are hearing each other and keeps other family members from interfering.

Parts are often better able than family members to resolve long-standing conflicts quickly and evolve new relationships when they finally face one another. This is because most polarized parts have never seen one another as they really are; instead, they are usually isolated from one another and vie to influence or overtake the Self. While isolated, each part maintains extreme ideas about or images of the other(s), which are confirmed consistently by the other part's (or parts') extreme behavior.

Some of these ideas or images will change as one part watches the Self interact with its counterpart (a part with whom it is polarized) through the room technique described above. Thus, the room technique, in addition to improving the relationship between the Self and a part, sets the stage for bringing polarized parts together. In less polarized systems, this preliminary stage of giving each polarized part individual attention is not necessary, and all the parts can simply join one another in a room as they emerge. In highly polarized internal systems, however, the room technique is an important first step toward harmonizing the system.

In highly polarized systems, before bringing two parts together, it is wise to ask each whether it would be willing to talk to the other in the presence of the Self. The Self can reassure each that he or she can keep the other from becoming disrespectful or hurtful; the Self can indeed do this if he or she remains differentiated. The Self can also tell each part what he or she has learned about the other's real nature, and can describe how much better things could be for each part if it could get along with the other.

When the parts agree to meet, the therapist has the client's Self bring the two parts together, get them to face each other, and have them interact concerning how they might improve their relationship. The Self may want to preface their dialogue with a statement such as "I know you both have in common that you want something good for all of us; you just differ in what it is or how to get it," or "Your battles are unnecessary and self-defeating. I want you to talk about how you can help each other, or at least get along differently." In this way, the Self becomes a therapist to the parts, and the therapist acts as an observing cotherapist. The Self reports on how the two parts are doing as they interact; the therapist gives advice or support, but mainly tries to keep the client's Self differentiated.

In many cases, the two parts begin a dialogue that moves along well on its own, with minimal input from the Self. At other times, one or both parts is recalcitrant, remaining extreme and not trying to discuss issues in good faith. The Self should firmly insist that the recalcitrant part or parts be respectful and that each should at least listen to the other part. Sometimes these efforts by the Self do not bear fruit, and nothing gets resolved in the initial meeting. When this is the case, each recalcitrant part may need more individual work, or the parts may simply need to meet repeatedly until they can trust enough not to be extreme in each other's presence.

Once the polarization between two parts begins to resolve, the Self may ask how they want to relate each other outside of these meetings. It is not uncommon to find dramatic reversals of relationships; for example, a critical manager that formerly hated a child exile may become a role model for or mentor of the child. The Self may also ask more questions about other parts that have been allied with one or the other side in the polarization, and may bring in these other parts to depolarize in a similar way.

In this way, with polarized internal systems, meeting individually with each part gradually changes to dyadic therapy with two parts, which in turn becomes internal group or family therapy. As mentioned earlier, the initial stages are not necessary for less polarized internal systems, where internal family therapy often can begin in the first session.

After a certain amount of depolarization of dyads or alliances has occurred, the Self may simply meet on a regular basis with the whole group (or at least with the parts that have been identified thus far or that respond to the Self's invitation to convene). To do this, the Self asks for the group to assemble and then asks questions about the state of the group. In the family therapy literature, these have been called "circular questions" (Tomm, 1985, 1987, 1988). Here are some examples:

- Who is the most upset? Who has been taking the most leadership?
- Who has been helping whom? Who is in conflict with whom?
- What do the parts think needs to happen today?

Through conversations with the group about questions like these, the goals for each session will emerge. I am frequently amazed at how this group, once somewhat depolarized, knows just what it needs and can convey that information to the Self. The Self simply tries to organize things so that the group's game plan can be implemented. Thus, if they say that one part is still extreme and needs a new role, the Self can interview that part in front of the group, and then can ask the group members for their reactions and for help in maintaining the negotiated change. If the problem is a disagreement between two parts, then the Self asks the two to face each other and works with them while the rest of the group watches.

As this kind of work in front of the group takes place, the Self can monitor the reaction of other parts to the work, because they are all there together. Afterwards the Self asks the group:

- Who was most upset by this work?
- Who might be inclined to interfere with it?
- Who is willing to try to help keep it going?

Much as in external family therapy, the goal is to get parts not only to resolve polarizations, but also to reorganize their relationships so that they all work together and help one another. In other words, the goal is not only to depolarize the parts, but also to balance and harmonize the entire internal system.

Thus, when a part needs help in changing, the Self asks for volunteers and discusses with the group how the help will be given. If the client faces a problem, the Self chairs a discussion with the whole group (or at least with those parts most interested in or knowledgeable about the problem), and a plan that involves the cooperation of various parts is devised to address the problem. If the client faces a big decision, the Self convenes the group and asks which parts favor one course of action and which the other. The Self moderates a debate over which way to go, and then, after listening to each side's case, makes the decision. The Self then asks those parts that "lost" in the decision what they might need to help them through the changes. In other words, the person becomes like a well-functioning social group that pools resources, debates decisions, and trusts its leadership.

Another amazing aspect of this internal family therapy is the amount of work that is accomplished by the group of parts on its own, often without the awareness of the Self. The Self may meet with the group to try to accomplish something, only to find that the parts have already carried it out and are working on other issues. Thus, the Self does not have to be with the parts for changes to occur; indeed, in many cases most of the change happens within the group, apart from the Self. When this kind of internal group process is achieved or already exists, psychotherapy can move very rapidly, because the client is able to use all of his or her resources to deal with problems.

Direct Access

In addition to in-sight, a therapist can work with a client's internal system in a different way. It is possible for the therapist to talk to parts of the client directly. It is also possible for the therapist to watch parts talking to one another or to the Self, rather than having that process described to him or her by the client, as is the case with in-sight. I call this mode "direct access" because the therapist is working with parts directly. This way of working with people was pioneered by Gestalt therapists, who would ask to talk to parts of a client or, in using the open-chair technique, would have two parts talk to each other by having the client shift between two chairs.

When I was first exploring internal systems, I relied heavily on direct access because I did not know about in-sight. In some sessions, a client would be hopping among five or six chairs as he or she brought internal dialogues to the surface. As I discovered the possibility of in-sight, I found that for most clients and for many purposes, it was more efficient and effective than direct access. Direct access still has some advantages over in-sight, however, and for the small number of clients who have difficulty experiencing inner vision, it is the primary way they can enter their inner worlds. At this point, then, there are some cases in which I use direct access as the primary mode, many cases in which I use it for certain purposes, and some cases in which I use in-sight exclusively. The reasons for this will become clearer after I describe the advantages of direct access.

First, direct access allows for a personal relationship to develop between a part and the therapist. When using in-sight, the therapist is always talking to the Self about what is happening, and consequently remains somewhat removed from the parts. In many people, however, certain parts need to experience the therapist directly, so that they feel reassured that he or she is competent and caring. In some cases this reassurance can only be derived by talking to the therapist directly.

Sometimes a client has been hurt or scared so badly in the past that the parts have very little trust in the Self. With such a client—for example, a survivor of severe and chronic incest—the therapist may have to be the Self for the client's system at first. That is, when it becomes clear that a client's parts will not cooperate with the Self, I have learned that continuing to expect and insist that the Self take the lead frustrates all members of the system. I have found that if I talk directly to each part and help resolve polarizations among them, much as the Self does during in-sight as described above, then I can also gradually help the parts appreciate the leadership potential of the Self.

Thus, in such a case, I begin as the Self for the system and spend much of each session talking directly to one part or another, or having two parts talk to each other. This work looks similar to that described in the literature on MPD. However, it differs from MPD work in this respect: As the parts begin to trust me, I suggest that they can also trust the Self and I increasingly shift responsibility to the Self, particularly for tasks between sessions.

This way of working can be very rewarding, because a therapist gets to know parts quite intimately; often, however, it is also quite challenging or frustrating, because some parts will deliberately try to provoke the therapist. With highly polarized clients, a therapist should only attempt direct access if the therapist is able to keep his or her own Self in the lead in the face of powerful provocation. When the therapist cannot keep an extreme part from overtaking his or her Self, he or she should admit this to the client and apologize. Particularly with direct access, if the therapist tries to cover up during or after a time when a part has taken over, the client's parts will sense this coverup and will trust the therapist less.

With other clients, the direct-access method complements the in-sight work. In many cases, before I use in-sight at all, I will talk directly to a client's managerial parts about what I plan to do and how safe it is. This way, these parts can check me out directly before opening up their system to me. After I have their permission, I may shift to in-sight for a period and then use direct access in special circumstances. For example, I will ask to speak to a part when the client's Self is having difficulty or when the therapy would be expedited by personal contact between the part and my Self.

In addition to permitting a personal relationship between the therapist and client's parts, the second advantage of direct access is that it offers the therapist and the client an often dramatic view of these inner personalities and their relationships. The sometimes amazing shifts in tone of voice, posture, and movement that take place when a part emerges provides compelling evidence of its existence. To watch a client shifting dramatically between two parts, saying things that the client didn't know he or she thought, often impresses even skeptical therapists sufficiently that they begin to see value in working with the multiplicity phenomenon. It also provides a visual picture of a part or of the relationship between parts, which can help the therapist understand and clarify the system and the individuals within it. I often recommend that students do nothing but direct access (with less polarized clients) for a period of time, because it is a good way to become familiar with the territory, especially if the students process information visually.

Direct access also sometimes allows parts to express themselves more fully than is possible through in-sight. As the therapist interviews a part, the part itself is frequently surprised to learn what it feels or thinks. Parts often value these opportunities for sanctioned external expression, and feel better understood by and connected to the listener.

Finally, the therapist is able to intervene directly in the relationship between two parts when they are interacting in front of him or her. For marital or family therapists, this is particularly appealing and familiar. As parts interact, with the client shifting from one chair to the next, it is like doing family or couples therapy, with the same intense emotional exchanges and the same role for the therapist.

The primary disadvantage of direct access is that, generally speaking, it is less efficient than in-sight. I can generally accomplish twice as much in an in-sight session as I could have if I had tried to do the same thing through direct access. This is particularly true for doing internal family therapy—working with the whole group as described above. In addition, direct access can be more dangerous with highly polarized clients because the therapist can inadvertently give access to parts that other parts may have struggled for years to keep hidden. If the therapist works carefully with such a system's managers, this danger can be avoided. But there is often a strong temptation to go a little further and talk to parts before the system is ready to tolerate their expression.

With highly polarized clients, there are inevitably times when some of these exiled parts break through and overtake the clients. One such client may call in the middle of the night in a panic, with scary thoughts or memories. Another may suddenly turn into a sobbing, desperate child in the middle of a session. Still another may begin shouting, becoming rageful and out of control. If the therapist can maintain Self-leadership, such a breakthrough can become an opportunity to demonstrate to a client's protective parts that his or her Self and/or the therapist's Self can help or deal with the part breaking through without being overwhelmed by it or by parts that are scared of it. Again, the importance of the therapist's maintaining Self-leadership in such situations cannot be overemphasized.

Directly accessing parts of clients is not difficult, and I have encountered few people who could not give access to their managerial parts, at least. Generally, these managers are nearby even in the first interaction between a therapist and client. Often the therapist is talking to them anyway when talking to the client, so the shift in acknowledging that you are talking directly to them is not a big one. For other, more remote parts, the shift is greater, so it may take longer before they are found or emerge.

The procedure is simple and, again, begins with the client focusing internally. The therapist asks the client to focus on a part, however he or she experiences it, and to ask whether it would be willing to speak directly to the therapist. If the part agrees, then the subsequent exchange may resemble the following:

THERAPIST: Okay, let the part speak through your mouth, as if the part is here and you are sitting over there, watching. In other words, don't blend with the part as it comes forward, but just watch or listen to my interaction with it.

MARY: I'll try, but I'm not sure if it will work.

THERAPIST: Don't try to think of what the part might say—just let it come out. I'll ask questions that will help it get going. If it doesn't happen, that's okay. We'll do something else. Are you ready?

MARY: I guess so.

THERAPIST: (*to Mary's part*) Okay, so what is it that you say to Mary?

MARY'S PART: I tell her not to trust anyone.

By asking a question about the part's relationship with Mary, the therapist in this case ensured a differentiated answer; that is, the part had to speak about itself as separate from her. Thus, the first questions should be relationship-focused. It can be phrased in one of these ways:

- What is it that you say or do to [client's name]?
- What do you make [client's name] do or think?
- How do you feel toward [client's name]?
- How do you think [client's name] feels toward you?
- Why do you do or say that to [client's name]?

After the part gives a differentiated answer (e.g., "I do _____ to Mary"), the therapist proceeds to ask the same kinds of questions discussed in the section on in-sight: questions concerning the part's relationship with other parts, with the Self, or with the therapist; its real intentions and desired new role; or ways in which it could be better cared for. After some progress has been made, the therapist suggests that he or she is ready to talk to the Self again, and may ask whether the part wants to add anything before that happens. The therapist should thank the part for coming forward and then ask to talk to the Self again.

The therapist then asks the client how that was for him or her to do. Most clients will respond that it was interesting, but some will say that it was very weird. They might worry that they are suffering from MPD or schizophrenia. It helps to re-emphasize that multiplicity is normal and that everyone can do this.

I have been discussing how direct access works when a therapist talks to a client's parts directly. The therapist can also observe a dialogue between a client's Self and a part. To do this, the therapist first accesses the client's part and tells it to imagine that the Self is sitting in a chair opposite it. The part is asked to say something to the Self (in the empty chair), after which the client moves into the empty chair and responds to the part's statement as the Self. In this way, the client moves back and forth between chairs, speaking as the part and then the Self, as long as is necessary to make some progress in their relationship. During this kind of dialogue, I usually try to remain as inactive as possible, limiting my role to ensuring that the Self maintains enough differentiation for the dialogue to progress. As with in-sight, I may initially have to facilitate the dialogue by suggesting questions for each to ask the other, or by ensuring that each is hearing the other; I then gradually reduce my activity. The goal is always for the Self to take leadership as quickly as possible.

The same basic procedure holds for creating a dialogue between two parts, or among several. After parts have been accessed, they are assigned chairs, and the client moves from one to another. Some clients do not have to move from chair to chair to differentiate parts; instead, such a client can remain in the same chair, making slight postural shifts as he or she shifts parts. The therapist works with the dialoguing parts in much the same way as with external family members. As soon as possible, the client's Self should be included in these interactions as well, and ideally takes the role of therapist to the dialoguing parts.

Cautions for Doing Inner Work Safely

Working with Recalcitrant Parts

After any period of direct access or in-sight, the therapist should end by asking to talk to the client's Self, so that the client leaves the office with the Self in the lead. Occasionally, with a highly polarized client, a part will not relinquish control and refuses to let the Self return. This is often

frightening for both therapist and client, but it is not necessarily dangerous. If possible, the therapist should get the part to talk about why it wants
to remain in control, and discuss whether or not those reasons are valid.
It is usually a mistake to try to coerce a part into relinquishing control; it
is often better to let the client leave with the part in charge than to enter
into a power struggle over the issue.

     This situation can be dangerous—mainly, when the therapist has
disregarded the signals from protective managers regarding the pace of
therapy and has prematurely allowed access to exiled parts. If this is the
case, the part in control will be either an enraged manager, a formerly
exiled part that fears being exiled again, or a desperate firefighter trying
to get out of the session as quickly as possible.

     To a manager, the therapist should apologize for endangering the
system and reassure the part that it will be consulted in the future. To an
exiled part, the therapist tries to provide assurance that the therapy is
designed to guarantee their release from exile eventually, and that the
part's current recalcitrance will only convince managerial parts that it
must remain exiled. The key is for the therapist to maintain Self-leadership
and convey respect for and awareness of the part's fears or pain, even in
the face of its extremes. When the part seems to listen to these reassurances, even if it remains extreme and in control, it is likely that the
therapist will get another chance. Sometimes a part will be willing to
discuss its real feelings only after being able to demonstrate that it can
take total control.

     On a very few occasions, I have not had time to say these things to
the part because the part makes the client bolt suddenly from my office.
Although this is very disconcerting (especially the first time it happens),
if the therapist has generated some credibility and good faith with the
client's Self and other parts, the client will eventually recontact the
therapist and amends can be made. Danger exists when the therapist has
only a tenuous relationship with the rest of the client's internal system, or
the therapist's parts have become extreme and provoked the client's parts.
In such an instance, the client may develop a general perception of
hopelessness or betrayal that can lead to severe consequences. The
therapist, with his or her Self in the lead, should try to recontact the client
as soon as possible and keep a dialogue going with the part in charge.

     Such episodes often arouse fears of self-destructive or suicidal behav-
ior in client and therapist alike, particularly when the part in charge is
threatening or hinting at such behaviors. As noted in Chapter 4, firefighters use apparently self-destructive behaviors (bulimia, self- cutting, drug
or alcohol abuse, extreme sexual behavior, or stealing) to release pressure
and avoid pain. In some ways, these behaviors can be seen as self-preserv-
ing; that is, they are attempts to protect rather than destroy the internal

system. They are not effective attempts, however, because in addition to their obvious physical consequences for the clients they activate other parts that attack the person for behaving destructively, thereby escalating inner polarizations.

Thus, if the therapist can see these behaviors this way and can maintain Self-leadership in the face of them or the threat of them, the client will not be as afraid of the parts that use them and will be better able to differentiate. This is not to say that the behaviors should be ignored or minimized by the therapist and client. Instead, they can be discussed as indications of the client's distress and opportunities to discover precisely what work needs to be done.

These firefighter behaviors may also increase, whether deliberately or inadvertently, as the formerly exiled hurt parts are given more access. The therapist can access the firefighters and ask about their reasons. If the therapist is compassionate and persistent, usually these parts will disclose their own pain or the pain of parts they are protecting. It is important to remember, however, that until the pain is dealt with differently, these firefighters will have trouble controlling their automatic reactions. Frequently, however, once a firefighter is reassured that the work with the exiles is safe and once it is depolarized with shaming managers, the firefighter becomes willing to negotiate how it reacts. It can agree to use a less dangerous and scary form of dissociation, or it might lower the intensity of its reaction. In general, firefighters need hope of change. If the therapist or the client's Self can give them hope, they become far less dangerous.

All this is not to imply that there is no danger when these parts take control. I find that the danger, however, lies less in the parts themselves than in the context in which they emerge. That is, if the external people or internal parts around these firefighters react in denying, shaming, coercive, or fearful ways, the danger increases. Any of these reactions can trigger an escalation of polarizations, so that the firefighters increase their protective behavior to the point that they become seriously destructive.

In a case where the person's external environment is seriously escalating the problem and is out of the therapist's control, or where a firefighter has taken the person into serious danger and deactivating it may take time, the therapist and client may want to consider a brief hospital stay. One goal of the hospitalization is to provide a safe, nurturing environment in which to do the internal work. Another goal is to provide a respite from the external polarizations, so that exiles can be addressed without the specter of dangerous firefighters making everyone frantic. The problem is that the orientation of many psychiatric hospital units has the opposite effect: Such units react to a firefighter's symptoms with coercion, overmedication, and pathologizing labels. This approach can further scare and disempower a client and external family, and can exacerbate their polarizations. In addition, particularly if the client has a history of having been coercively abused, parts of the client will be terrified to go into any context where authorities again have so much power over him or her. For all these reasons, the consequences of hospitalization should be thoroughly considered, and an effort should be made to find a program that is compatible with the IFS approach.

Acknowledging the Nature of Parts

A final danger relates to the nature of the parts. My understanding of what the parts are has evolved considerably over the years of doing this work, and undoubtedly will continue to evolve. When I first began working this way, I came from a constructivistic orientation, so I thought I was cocreating the inner dialogues with clients rather than uncovering something that was there. That is, I thought clients were responding to subtle clues from me and were imagining that these parts operated in ways that we created in our interaction.

It gradually became clear that although my questioning or mood had some impact on the system, these inner personalities had a life of their own as well and could not be simply imagined. I shifted to the position that perhaps these were unidimensional mental states, each designed for a certain valuable role.

As described in earlier chapters, as I have become better acquainted with parts, they have taught me to view them multidimensionally—as if they were people at different ages and with different talents (even though they do not always appear that way at first during in-sight). That is, each part has a full range of feelings, needs, and desires, which correspond to its age, gender, and innate characteristics or talents—just like external people.

The mind's natural multiplicity is a difficult proposition for many therapists to accept—it took me many years to come to this position. The idea that we are a collection of people does not fit well with our Western scientific tradition. It is not necessary to see parts this way to have success with the model; indeed, many therapists using it today hold a constructivistic or "mental states" view.

The danger, however, is that in viewing parts in the more limited, "mental states" way, therapists will underestimate and underrespond to them. That is, in this book I often use one- or two-word descriptions or names to refer to parts (e.g., an achievement part, a child-like part, or a protective parts; the Achiever, the Little Girl/Boy, or the Protector, etc.). When I saw parts as mental states, I believed that such a description or name adequately captured a part, because I saw it as having a limited set of feelings or thoughts and as being designed for a limited role.

Now I have learned that parts are not *just* protecting or achieving or sad or angry parts, even though they may be functioning in those limited ways within the internal system. For example, an angry part may also have scared, sad, sexual, or happy feelings. Perhaps the part has been taking the role of the Angry One to protect other parts or because it is exiled, but it is far more that just an angry part. It is often an adolescent.

Whether a therapist views parts as "real" has two implications for internal work. The first has to do with what the angry part will need to change. Since it is a teenager and not just a mental state, it does not just need to be calmed out of its angry condition. In all likelihood, it will also need to be talked to about its hurt or about the way the world works. It will need to see that the Self and other parts care for and appreciate it. It will need what a lonely or hostile adolescent needs in order to feel a sense of belonging and security.

The second implication has to do with the ultimate role a part takes. Perhaps this angry teenager is well suited to the role of helping the client assert himself or herself, and so it may choose to remain in the role of the Asserter (sometimes the Angry Asserter), even after it has been harmoniously integrated into the larger group. It may, on the other hand, choose an entirely different role, perhaps to give the person sensitivity regarding the feelings of others. If a therapist sees it as just a mental state, the therapist will be less interested in helping the part discover the best role for itself, based on its feelings, talents, and desires.

Thus, if the therapist views parts simply as mental states or as introjected images, he or she will relate to them differently than the therapist who sees them as people. It is possible to view them as people while one works with the internal system, but to think about them in other ways that are less disconcerting when one is theorizing. The important thing is that when one is relating to them, their personhood must be respected.

I still use one- or two-word descriptions or labels for parts, but now these refer to the roles or images the client finds the parts enacting, rather than to their essence or something inherent in their nature. The roles or images with which parts eventually wind up may be entirely unrelated to the ones with which they started. It is important to remind clients to change names for parts as the original names become unsuitable.

Conclusion

In this chapter I have tried to provide directions for the technical side of IFS work with individual clients, as well as guidelines for doing this work safely. Out of fear of selling this model "before its time" (R. C. Schwartz

& Perrotta, 1985), I have waited many years before publishing this material on technique. I wanted to be sure I knew enough of the dangers and how to deal with them to ensure that therapists would not hurt clients by using the model. I believe that its time has finally come. (Appendix A provides a summary outline of the steps described in this chapter and in Chapter 4.)

As a therapist, you, the reader, will reach internal impasses and scary moments in doing IFS work with clients. Parts of you will lobby for discarding this model and returning to methods with which you feel competent; this happens to many therapists when they begin using the model. To counter this tendency, it helps to talk to colleagues who know something about the model or are trying to explore it too. In addition, try as best you can to keep your Self in the lead, even in the face of blind alleys or extreme parts of your client or yourself. Finally, trust your client's Self and parts to help you learn how to help him or her. Even in a case where it may not seem so, the internal family ultimately knows best.

CHAPTER 6

The Model's Views of Families

The IFS model views families in the same way it views individuals. Families carry burdens, polarize into the three-group structure described earlier (exiles, managers, and firefighters), exhibit imbalances, and have leadership problems. Thus, it is possible to use the same conceptual map that one uses to understand individuals to understand families.

In addition, the goals for working at the external level are the same as those for internal work. At the internal level, one primary goal is to release parts from their extreme roles so that they can adopt their preferred, valuable roles in harmony with one another. This is also a primary goal for families: to release family members from their extreme roles so that they can adopt their preferred, harmonious roles. The constraints that keep family members and parts in these extreme roles are also the same at both levels.

This chapter uses the IFS principles introduced in Chapter 1—development, balance, harmony, and leadership—to help in understanding family process.* The reader should bear in mind, of course, that these principles apply to human systems at all levels and can be translated easily to other levels. I also suggest how these four principles are interrelated—how each can constrain or enhance the others.

To illustrate one way in which these dimensions can constrain one another, let's look at the impact of patriarchal attitudes on a family. When a family adopts the burden of patriarchy from its culture (which involves the dimension of family development), the males in the family will have more influence and resources and less domestic (but more economic) responsibility than the females (imbalance), which in turn will create chronic resentments and conflicts (disharmony or polarization). In these conflicts, the parents will side with the males, giving them more oppor-

---

*I am indebted to discussions with Peter Thomas for clarifying these ideas.

tunities (biased leadership); these biases, to complete the circle, reinforce the patriarchal attitude.

Concomitantly, an improvement in any of these dimensions can affect the other three. For example, if a therapist helps this patriarchal family to balance influence, responsibilities, and resources, its leadership will have to become less biased. After an initial backlash, this improved family balance and leadership will gradually create more harmony, and the family members will have to confront their patriarchal attitudes.

Now let me highlight parallels across levels of human systems by focusing on the internal system of one member of that family, to show how her inner life resembles her family's structure. The burden of patriarchy (development) leads the adolescent daughter to overvalue her striving, approval-seeking parts and to devalue her sensitive, caring parts (imbalance). These dominant approval-seeking parts are constantly disdainful of the "weakness" of the sensitive parts (polarization), and the daughter's Self allows the dominant parts to run her life (biased leadership) in order to keep her safe and competitive. This inner system is approved of by her patriarchal family and culture, because it produces good grades and demure behavior. This approval reinforces her patriarchal burden, despite the price she pays in terms of inner conflict and, in this case, bulimia.

The following sections of this chapter describe these four dimensions in more depth, beginning with development and moving to balance, harmony, and leadership.

Development

Family therapy has always been ambivalent at best about exploring a family's history or development. The field was born in part as a reaction against the psychodynamic emphasis on early childhood development. Some attempts have been made to consider the tasks involved in each stage of the family's life cycle and to incorporate that thinking into family systems theory (e.g., Carter & McGoldrick, 1989); by and large, however, the systems-oriented schools of family therapy have remained present-focused. Another reason for this is that family therapy applied biological and mechanical systems thinking to families. That kind of systems thinking is more concerned with how machines or biological systems operate in the present than in how they have developed. A mechanic who tries to fix a machine is concerned with finding the problem in the way it functions now. History is not terribly relevant to the mechanic, because no matter how the machine was broken, the solutions will be the same.

When I began working with people's intrapsychic systems, I believed that I could reorganize their internal families' present functioning without much consideration of their development. The more I worked with people's internal families, however, the more I came to appreciate the impact of historical constraints.

Sustaining and Constraining Environments

Although I believe that most human systems come fully equipped, in that they have all the resources they need at the outset for a healthy, harmonious existence, they need time within a sustaining environment to develop those resources. The members of a system need time to discover their visions and preferred roles; to harmonize their relationships; and to balance influence, resources, responsibilities, and boundaries. The system's leaders also need time to establish credibility, trust, and a shared vision. If the system exists in a sustaining, nurturing environment during its development, this healthy state will unfold naturally and at its proper pace. Indeed, central to the IFS model is the belief that systems have a wisdom about this pace, which needs to be respected.

If instead a system develops within a polarized, constraining environment, its resources will be less accessible. It is thus more likely to become structurally unbalanced and polarized, with problematic leadership. In other words, the system is likely to reflect the imbalanced and polarized systems in which it is embedded, because these qualities tend to be contagious.

Like ideas pertaining to the other three principles—balance, harmony, and leadership—these ideas regarding development apply to humanity at all levels. From a child to a family, from a company to a country, a human system needs time in a sustaining environment for healthy development. I do not subscribe, however, to the concept that a single critical period spent in a constraining environment destroys or severely curtails the system's chances for health. No matter how early in its development a human system has been constrained—whether by abuse, neglect, and deprivation, or by being subjected to extreme values, responsibilities, or trauma—it still contains an undamaged, fully capable Self that can restore some level of balance and harmony once the constraints are released. In addition, the members of the system, no matter how polarized and extreme, want to return to valuable roles and will do so when they believe it is safe. Thus, the harmonious development or reorganization of a human system can take place at any point in the system's life.

In addition, healthy development does not necessarily require great amounts of time or outside intervention. I do not believe that a human system must pass through a series of crucial stages in sequence to achieve maturity, with the implication that if a stage is missed, the system has to return to it and then proceed sequentially through the remaining stages. Instead, the release of the system's resources for effective leadership is often enough to generate "virtuous cycles" (balancing and harmonizing sequences—the opposite of "vicious cycles"), so that the system rapidly heals itself. Before these resources can be released in some cases, however, imbalances and polarizations must be dealt with, and the members need time to build trust in the leadership.

Also, in some cases a system must be released from the grip of its history. This section on development focuses on historical constraints— that is, on the impediments to a system's healthy organization as it developed. These constraints often take the form of extreme beliefs or feelings, which, after being injected into the system, remain to govern many aspects of its functioning. The family therapy field has called these constraints family "myths" or "rules"; in the IFS model, they are called "burdens." A family or a person can accrue burdens from a variety of sources, including trauma, the family of origin, or the culture.

Burdens Created by Trauma

Trauma can have a highly deleterious effect on human systems, especially while they are developing. Over the past several years I, like growing numbers of therapists, have worked extensively with adult survivors of childhood sexual abuse (R. C. Schwartz, 1992; Goulding & Schwartz, in press). These clients have taught me a great deal about the effects of trauma on internal systems. These effects can be extrapolated to families.

It is a common assumption that surviving trauma builds character. This is the case however, only when the system's leadership remains strong throughout the trauma, protecting and comforting vulnerable members. When that occurs, trauma does build character in the sense of increasing trust in and respect for leadership. One goal of the IFS model is to help systems develop this kind of leadership, so that any future traumas will be character-building rather than character-destroying. Thus, trauma can have two main constraining effects: (1) The system's leaders either abdicate, are protected (hidden), or are discredited, resulting in attempts to lead by ill-equipped members; and (2) some parts of the system become burdened and frozen in time at the point of the trauma, and consequently are exiled or left behind.

Thus, the effect of a trauma on a family will depend at least in part on how the leaders behave during and after it. If the trauma involves physical danger or injury and the parents are able to protect the family, maintaining Self-leadership and dealing effectively with injuries, then they gain respect and trust. Similarly, if the trauma involves painful loss and the parents are able to comfort and nurture the suffering members,

perpetrators

again they gain stature. On the other hand, if the parents are themselves overcome with grief, fear, or pain and consequently abdicate, or if they stoically deny or minimize a child's or children's feelings, they lose trust and respect.

In cases where parents abdicate, children often have to protect, comfort, or distract parents or handle the family, leaving these youngsters with the burdens of overresponsibility and protectiveness. In these protective roles, some children are forced to exile their own hurt or scared parts, and to elevate their managers. Other children may feel compelled to distract the family from their crisis with firefighter activity. Not only does remaining in these manager and firefighter roles leave children carrying young parts full of fear and pain from the trauma itself; these parts are also abandoned and isolated within the child, compounding the effects of the trauma.

In this way, trauma can create the three-group polarization (exiles, managers, and firefighters) within family members as well as within the family. Family members often become locked into the extreme roles that they were forced into by the trauma. They also live in fear of the emergence of exiles within each family member that remain frozen at the point of the trauma. Some family members may become dominated by parts that are frozen at the time of the trauma; as a result, they have difficulty functioning. They may be so wrought with grief, fear, or guilt that they bother others in the family who are trying to forget and move on. They can become family exiles, sometimes being exiled literally to residential placements or foster homes.

It is not just the hurt, vulnerable family members who are exiled in traumatized families. When there is a perpetrator of the trauma, frequently the members who are enraged at the perpetrator advocate action or revenge rather than passivity. They may threaten family managers, and become exiled. Or those who blame the leaders for not protecting the family are stifled or exiled.

Often, however, it is not people who are exiled in families, but the feelings or topics related to the trauma. These become the family secrets about which everyone is aware but no one speaks. The family members are all trying to exile the parts of them that are stuck in the traumatic time, and fear that these related feelings or topics will trigger those parts.

Burdens Created by Constraining Environments

Some people or families never experience severe trauma, and yet they become highly imbalanced and polarized because of developing within an imbalanced and polarized system—that is, within a constraining environment. As it develops, a human system is highly dependent on its environment for survival, and consequently is eager to be valued by that environment. As discussed previously, a young child cannot survive alone and consequently is highly dependent on his or her parents. The child believes, often correctly, that the penalty for parents' not valuing or caring about him or her may be abandonment, severe harm, or death. As a result, a child becomes very sensitive to messages from parents regarding their evaluation of him or her.

Where those messages are consistently reassuring, this hypersensitivity abates quickly, and the child's system is not constrained by this burden of worry from developing harmoniously. In a constraining environment, however, the child is likely to receive inconsistent messages at best regarding his or her worth during this period of high dependence. When a child is uncertain or pessimistic about his or her value, the child strives to discern and become what is perceived as pleasing to the parents. In this approval-craving state, parts of a child imitate one or both parents in an effort to make the child what the parent wants. These parts take on the burden of perfectionism or disapproval, becoming internalized critical parents. This process has been called "internalization" or "introjection" in other intrapsychic models.

Families go through a similar internalizing process during their development. In mainstream U.S. culture, families are valued by how "functional" they are. That is, a family's success is measured by how independent, productive, and attractive its members are—how well they fit into and contribute to the mainstream. Most families in the United States depend on the mainstream culture for their survival. As a result, family members internalize U.S. middle-class burdens of striving toward achievement, perfect appearance, and isolating autonomy. These burdens lead to family imbalances, disharmony, and leadership problems, and to vicious cycles among those three dimensions.

Legacy Burdens

When two people marry and start a family, the genes each carries will govern many aspects of the family's life and appearance. Similarly, both spouses bring burdens to the family, which will also have a large impact on the family's life. Some of these burdens were accrued from each spouse's respective family of origin. Events or interactions that occurred during the spouse's childhood can leave parts of the spouse carrying burdens. Some families have passed burdens from generation to generation—burdens that were first instilled hundreds of years earlier. One or both spouses may be the carrier of a legacy-like burden, such as shame, perfectionism, powerlessness, rage, great expectations, or any number of other extreme ideas or emotions.

The cross-generational transferral of burdens is a natural outgrowth of polarization within parents, because children will often relate to their parts in the same way that their parents related to those parts. In addition, a parent will relate to a child, when the child acts like one of the parent's parts, in the same way the parent relates to that part. In this sense, then, internal relationships, as well as burdens, are passed across the generations.

As an example, let us return to the case of Sally (see Chapter 2). Sally's father hated weakness inside and outside him. He was dominated by stoic, critical parts and was ashamed of his own hurt parts. When Sally was a child, every time she was sad and cried, her father became agitated and impatient. As a result, Sally become impatient with her own sadness and tried to keep that sad part out of her life. Stoic, critical parts that disdained weakness came to dominate her in the same way they dominated her father. In this way, he passed on to her the legacy burden of stoicism.

A burden that is extreme in one direction, however, may often create the opposite extreme. When Sally reached adolescence, the hurt, needy exiles she had abandoned for years overwhelmed her. Her father tried again to shame them away, but that only increased their sense of worthlessness and desperation. Thus, her father not only passed on the burden of stoicism, but also the opposite burden of neediness and shame. As the proverb says, "You can drive the devil out of your garden, but you will find him again in the garden of your son." We generate in our children the burdened parts that dominate us, as well as the ones we demonize.

This process of passing on burdens is not limited to families. Whole cultures can carry legacy burdens as the result of being massacred, colonized, enslaved, or impoverished. Or a culture may carry a burden such as patriarchy or racism, whose origins are less clearly traceable. Cultural burdens constrain all the families within the culture, and in turn burden the individuals within the families.

Developmental Burdens

Other burdens are accrued as a family goes through its own life cycle. Unexpected deaths or births can leave burdens of grief or resentment. Strained parent–child relationships can leave burdens of inadequacy, worthlessness, and rage. When parents are highly polarized with each other or are forced for some reason to abdicate their leadership, children are left with burdens of protecting a parent or of responsibility for the family. I work with many clients who were sexually abused as children by a parent. This abuse loads a child with a number of disabling burdens, from shame and worthlessness to rage and perfectionism.

Not all burdens are accrued from within the family. Family members may experience rejection, humiliation, or physical or sexual abuse from people outside the family, which may leave lasting burdens. Repeated encounters with racism, sexism, or classism can accumulate into back-breaking burdens.

Tangible Burdens

The burdens discussed above take the form of constraining attitudes or emotions. There are other, more tangible burdens that constrain families as the result of their socioeconomic context or, for lack of a better term, their fate. For example, having a chronically ill or disabled member taxes a family's economic and emotional resources. Resources are also drained by the burden of poverty: Family members have to work hard just to survive, have to live in dangerous communities, and receive few rewards.

Because of legacy or developmental burdens a family member already carries, he or she may react to a tangible burden in an extreme way that compounds its constraining effect. In addition, tangible burdens such as poverty and disabilities often put new emotional or attitudinal burdens on family members (e.g., hopelessness, inadequacy, or resentment), which also compound the impact of the tangible burden.

Balance

With physiological systems, balance is a crucial principle. To remain healthy, our bodies must maintain certain levels of blood sugar, acidity, and electrolytes. Imbalances in these variables may cause chronic degeneration of physiological systems or may prompt homeostatic responses from our bodies that can create problems.

Human systems also need to be balanced to remain healthy. Instead of blood sugar or electrolytes, however, the crucial variables are influence, resources, responsibilities, and boundaries. Burdens affect the balance of these variables within a family. I briefly discuss these four variables within families, and then describe the impact upon them of burdens and the problems or syndromes resulting from burdens.

Variables That Need to Be Balanced

In a family, "influence" refers to who makes major financial, educational, geographic, or other life style decisions, as well as decisions regarding division of resources and responsibilities. The family's "resources" include material resources (food, shelter, clothing, money), leisure time, rolodex

nurturance, attention, and guidance; they also include praise from parents and access to friends. "Responsibilities" within a family include rearing and nurturing children, generating income, developing and maintaining relationships and interests outside the nuclear family, and organizing and maintaining the home.

"Boundaries" are distinctions regarding what or who is included in and excluded from in a system. In some systems boundaries are relatively easy to define and agree upon. A car includes all those parts that travel with it. If we remove the horn, it is no longer part of the system of the car. If we put the horn back in, it is once again within the car's boundaries. With human systems, boundaries are not always so clear, and polarizations can arise over their definition.

Two decades ago, structural family therapists postulated that healthy families had clear boundaries around themselves and their subsystems (Minuchin, 1974). "Clear boundaries" (what I am calling "balanced boundaries") were defined as those that permitted appropriate access to other subsystems, but also protected a family system from intrusions that impeded its development. Problematic boundaries were either too diffuse, allowing too much access from other systems, or too rigid, allowing too little access. Thus in human systems, boundaries are rules regarding who has access to whom and how. A family functions best when each member is a part of the subsystems he or she needs to develop, and the boundaries around each subsystem are balanced between access and privacy.

Balance versus Equality

By asserting that these four variables need to be balanced, I am not suggesting that each member should at all times have equal influence, resources, or responsibilities, or that boundaries around subsystems should never be rigid or diffuse. People have different roles within a system. Ideally, a person's role will be determined by his or her age, ability, vision, temperament, and desire. People also have different needs, according to their roles and levels of development. Thus, parents in a family should have more influence and responsibility than their young children; the children will require more of certain resources (e.g., nurturance, free time, and guidance) than parents.

Within the same developmental level, however, some kind of equitable balance of these dimensions is important. For example, within the parental subsystem, neither husband nor wife should chronically have more influence, resources, or responsibilities than the other. The same is true for the young siblings. This is not to say that these variables need to be divided equally, such that, for example, both spouses do exactly the same housework or make the same amount of money. In addition, there may be periods during which imbalances are necessary—for example, when one spouse goes to school and the other has to support the family. This is not a problem if, later, the other spouse has the opportunity for imbalance in his or her direction.

A healthy family assesses the situation of each family member in regard to each of these variables—including in the equation such factors as the perceived tediousness of the responsibility, perceived value of the resource, and perceived importance of the sphere of influence—to see where chronic imbalances exist. The family members then discuss the source of any imbalances and how to correct them.

Imbalances Created by Burdens

Burdens create imbalances and impede a family's ability to correct them. For example, as described earlier, the burden of patriarchy creates a family in which the males in the family are given more influence and resources than the females. It also creates rigid boundaries between males and females. Many families struggle to shed the burden of patriarchy, but because we are embedded in a patriarchal society, this is difficult. As I discuss in Chapter 8, families tend to absorb the burdens and imbalances of the cultures in which they are embedded.

Some families of young female bulimic clients have absorbed from mainstream U.S. culture toxic doses not only of patriarchal burdens, but also of the burdens of perfect appearance and achievement. Such families are as dominated by these striving, competitive, and critical parts as are their bulimic daughters' intrapsychic worlds. Family members who are hurt by or cannot live up to the extreme standards imposed by these burdens become family exiles, much as the bulimic clients' sensitive, compassionate parts become internal exiles.

Imbalances Created by Problems or Syndromes

In many of these families, the bulimia (or other problem or syndrome) itself becomes a tangible burden that also creates imbalances. For example, a bulimic daughter often absorbs an inordinate amount of her parents' attention and time, leaving her siblings feeling neglected and resentful. Because of her syndrome, she may be excused from the responsibilities and pressures placed on her siblings, and she may gain more influence than the others over family decisions. Her siblings and one or both parents will react to the new family imbalance created by her syndrome.

Problems or syndromes do not always cause major family imbalances. The extent to which one member's problem creates imbalances in a family depends on aspects of the problem itself. That is, some problems are less draining, stigmatizing, guilt-generating, and intimidating than others. The degree of imbalance created by a problem will depend on the following:

1. How socially acceptable the problem is.
2. How much the family members can be implicated in its onset.
3. How much the family members believe the person can control it.
4. How dangerous or damaging they believe it to be.
5. How much hope they have that experts can solve it.
6. Whether they believe they can help deal with it and are clear about what they and the person need to do.
7. Whether the problem has a predictable course and they can know with some confidence when it is solved.
8. How much it drains resources or shifts responsibilities.

All these factors are another way of asking how burdening the problem is. That is, what kinds of emotional, cognitive, and tangible burdens does the problem carry, and how do those burdens affect the family's balance?

Given these considerations, the least burdening kind of problem would be one that is socially acceptable; of clear etiology unrelated to the person or family; only mildly dangerous, damaging, or draining; and treatable through expert intervention, with clear-cut roles for family members and for the person. Any number of illnesses fit this description, and thus generally do not create great imbalance within the family system. A problem that departs from this description in any of these respects has an increased potential to generate imbalances.

Unfortunately, bulimia strays from this depiction of the ideal problem in all of these respects. Consequently, bulimia has great potential for unbalancing families. It is a highly embarrassing, potentially dangerous syndrome with an unclear etiology and prognosis. Various family or parental characteristics have been put forth as being related to its onset, but it is also the kind of problem that makes the child's will power highly suspect. Since there is no consensus regarding state-of-the-art treatment, with clearly delineated roles for all involved, there is great potential for divisiveness as to the type of treatment and the behaviors of family members or the bulimic client. Its course may vary considerably, swinging between periods of improvement and discouraging relapse. It can drain family resources on several levels, particularly if parents engage in taxing and frustrating attempts to control it. Because of all these aspects of bulimia, it is more likely than many other problems to activate extreme parts of family members, leading to the imbalances described above.

Harmony

Whereas "balance" refers to the four system variables discussed above (resources, responsibilities, influence, and boundaries), "harmony" is used here to describe other qualities of relationships within a system. A number of terms have been used to describe relationships in well-functioning families—"cohesive," "flexible," "communicating effectively," "caring," "supportive," "cooperative," and "low in conflict," to name a few. All of these can be encapsulated by the dimension of harmony. In a harmonious family the members enjoy their roles, or at least understand the contribution of their roles and feel appreciated for them. The family is directed by a common vision that is understood and valued by everyone. In addition, individual differences among family members in vision and style are respected, and an attempt is made to find a fit between each individual's vision and that directing the family. Competition among members may exist, but it is contained by an underlying caring among the competitors, as well as by a commitment to the welfare of the system and to the larger ecology of systems in which they are embedded. Competition is not driven by fear, because the loser is not threatened with loss of status or role. All family members are willing to sacrifice some personal resources and goals, because they care about the other members and they understand and support the larger vision of the family. Communication is direct, spontaneous, and honest; as a result, conflicts are resolved and imbalances are corrected.

Harmonious families are highly sustaining for people. Once people have felt themselves a part of this shared harmony, thereafter they strive to regain it or feel its loss. If asked about the best times in their lives, many people speak longingly of high school, college, or military groups (or even street gangs); they feel isolated in their often fragmented nuclear families and jobs. People want to live in what I call "sustaining environments," but they have trouble finding them. Mobile, fear-driven, competitive U.S. mainstream culture is not conducive to the formation of harmonious companies, communities, extended families, nuclear families, or internal families. Instead, these often become "constraining environments," in which maintaining balance and harmony is more difficult.

Polarization

When families become heavily burdened or imbalanced, harmony is very difficult to maintain. Family members tend to polarize with one another, which is the opposite of harmony. In a polarized relationship, each person shifts from his or her harmonious position to a rigid, extreme position in opposition to or competition with another. Communication and caring between the polarized members break down as rigid boundaries build up. The members anticipate dire consequences if they retreat from their extreme positions; instead, they strive to maximize their influence and resources or to minimize their responsibilities, regardless of the effects of their behavior on others in the family.

Polarizations can constrain a family in several ways. First, each person in a polarized relationship is forced to maintain a position or role that he or she does not necessarily want or feel valued in. Second, the polarized roles can become so extreme as to be destructive to the whole family. Third, polarized people cooperate poorly and can become so resentful or competitive that they actively try to sabotage one another, or even the family itself.

Distraction

The fourth way in which polarizations can constrain a family merits extended discussion. The tension generated by polarized relationships can create the need for some kind of distraction. Everyone in the family fears the consequences of an escalation in the polarization; these might include the loss of privilege, harm or elimination of one member or another, or the disintegration of the whole system. This is particularly threatening when the family's leaders (commonly the parents) are polarized.

To avoid the feared escalation, family members may create distraction in a variety of ways. One or both of two polarized people may pull in a third member to take their side or fight their battles for them, generating destructive "coalitions." Or the two polarized people may shift their focus onto a third member, in either a scapegoating or a nurturing way. Or they may become obsessed with less threatening issues. Finally, other members of the system who are not involved in the polarization directly, but who are threatened by it, may create distraction with their behavior or problems.

Thus, a highly threatening polarization has a powerfully constraining effect on all members of the family. Fear of an escalation keeps the issues underlying the polarization from being discussed and resolved; in other words, it keeps those issues exiled. Everyone in the family may become so focused on the polarization, and involved in distracting from it, that the development of each member is constrained. For example, children can become so worried about their parents that they are not free to explore other relationships.

In addition, the members of a highly polarized family cannot adapt to changes in their development or in their environment. Instead, any change is threatening because it may disturb the family's precarious network of protective distractions and coalitions, leading to the feared escalation. Polarized systems become rigidly homeostatic, in that they tolerate only narrow ranges of behaviors and attitudes, and they react with strong sanctions to deviations. They also strongly resist the intervention of outsiders.

Family Exiles, Managers, and Firefighters

Once again a parallel between internal and external system emerges. Polarized external families organize in the same way as polarized internal families: with exiles, managers, and firefighters. In families, the exiles are the threatening and emotion-charged issues or secrets that everyone tries to avoid. They are also the extreme parts of family members that emerge in relation to those issues and secrets. These exiled issues and secrets vary from family to family, but they often center around past or current episodes when extreme angry or indulgent parts of various family members took over, hurting or scaring other members. Commonly exiled issues thus include extramarital affairs, alcohol or drug binges, angry rages, suicidal episodes, or other betrayals or abandonments. The family members fear the surfacing of these issues not only for the pain or embarrassment their memory brings, but also for the parts that might surface with them and might take over again.

To keep these issues hidden, some family members become managers, taking on the same roles as the managers in internal families. Some family managers try to control the content and flow of family communication, steering conversations away from feared topics. Some focus a family's attention on nonthreatening obsessions, such as achievement or perfect appearance. They enforce family rules against expressions of vulnerability or distress with criticism and shame. Others inject a variety of fears into the family so that no one takes risks. They pass on the legacy burden of low self-esteem, which keeps family members in their safe place.

Other family members are forced into firefighter roles, in parallel again to internal firefighters. Family firefighters react in extreme and impulsive ways to the underlying tension within the family. When that tension reaches threatening levels, they find either a way to distract the family's attention, or a way to numb or palliate the distressed family members; they put out or steer everyone clear of family fires. An acting-out child may be serving this firefighter function, but so are the parents who become obsessed with controlling the child and shift the conversation to the child's behavior whenever scary escalations begin. With bulimia, a client's syndrome can become a firefighter focus for the client's whole family. Yet many of these families were using food and eating to distract or palliate long before the clients became bulimic. In this sense, a client's syndrome is just an extension of a family's firefighter activity of choice.

This is not to imply that the persons in firefighter roles are aware that they are protecting other family members from a specific threatening issue. Instead, they may be simply reacting automatically to shifts in mood of the other family members. These shifts trigger firefighter parts within the persons that take over and protect them from their own exiled parts, while simultaneously protecting the other family members from exiled issues.

The Family's Need for a Distraction

The whole question of whether symptoms serve protective functions within families is a complex one; to avoid some common misconceptions, I discuss it further here. A cornerstone of early models of family therapy was the notion that symptoms are family distractions. Later, this functionalist notion was challenged and is now in disfavor within family therapy (Nichols & Schwartz, 1994). I believe that the early versions of this notion contained implications that contributed to the current backlash. These unfortunate implications included the following: (1) Symptoms or problems *always* serve protective functions in families; (2) the family function they serve is the primary reason for the symptoms' existence and should be the main focus of therapy; and (3) family members want the symptoms or problems so that they can be distracted.

The result of these implications was that therapists were forever searching for the putative family function of symptoms even when none existed. Therapists also ignored other aspects of their clients' inner or outer worlds because they were so fixated on the symptoms' function. They did not trust changes other than changes in families that, theoretically, made the symptoms less necessary. In addition, many parents were made to feel responsible for their children's problems, as if they would rather have their children suffer than face their own issues.

In contrast, the IFS model suggests that although some problems are serving firefighter functions within families, many are not. Presupposing such a role for a person or problem violates the spirit of the IFS model, in which the therapist and family or client explore constraints together, without presuming. In addition, even in a case where the problem does seem to lie in a distractive role, the IFS therapist does not assume that this role is necessarily the most powerful or important constraint, and thus, does not have to focus on it. Instead, the therapist and client/family are free to focus on any number of other constraints—a process that may create sufficient change for the person to be able to leave the firefighter role without its ever being mentioned.

Finally, when a client's or symptom's firefighter role does become the focus of IFS therapy, no family member, including the client, feels blamed for needing or wanting it. This is because the IFS model distinguishes between the person or family's need or desire for a distraction and need or desire for the problem. That is, the IFS model assumes that members of distressed human systems at any level will frequently need or want to be distracted from threatening problems. This is a normal and sometimes necessary reaction. To understand this process better, we need only reflect on a time when we were terrified to face something, believed that attempts to face it would be futile or make things worse, and thought that if it were ignored long enough it might go away. In such a predicament, we probably seized any opportunity to avoid the dreaded subject, and if other problems surfaced or were available, we became obsessed with them. We did not *want* these other problems, and did not know that by obsessing we were maintaining them or making them worse. We focused on them because they were there; they were available.

Fear-plagued families are no different from us. They become so desperate for a distraction from exiled issues that they will use anything for that purpose. If a client's bulimia is available as a distraction, family members may use it as one of many obsessive distractions. But the therapist must not conclude that they *want* the client to have bulimia so that they can be distracted. Instead, they strongly wish the client were healthy, but since this is not the case and the syndrome is there, they use it often without understanding that by using it they play a role in maintaining or exacerbating it.

Enmeshment   reciprocal role procedures

Thus far in this section on harmony, I have focused on polarized relationships. What about the smothering closeness that also characterizes relationships in many troubled human systems? This excessive closeness has been given a variety of labels, including "enmeshment," "fusion," and "symbiosis." People in such relationships report almost being able to feel each other's feelings, often speak for and protect each other, and overreact to each other's emotions. They have trouble separating from or differing with each other. This kind of enmeshment is seen as particularly destructive when it is cross-generational—that is, when it occurs between a parent and a child. The child is constrained from getting to know himself or herself as an individual and from forming other appropriate relationships; the child is also burdened with the need to please or take care of the parent. Complimentarily, the parent neglects his or her relationship with a partner or with friends.

Polarization and enmeshment are interrelated. Where one finds extreme or chronic polarization in a family, one is also likely to find people who are extremely close. This complementarity between polarization and enmeshment can also be viewed through the dimension of balance discussed above. That is, at either extreme, the boundaries in the relationship are imbalanced. Polarized relationships tend to have rigid boundaries, and enmeshed relationships tend toward diffuse boundaries.

Thus, enmeshment is a common consequence of polarization, and vice versa. When family members *A* and *B* are highly polarized, one or both will be inclined to become extremely close to another family member, *C*. Similarly, when *A* and *B* are very close, *C* may feel excluded and become polarized. In addition, there are many dyadic relationships that contain qualities of both enmeshment and polarization—the proverbial love–hate relationships. In such a case, some parts of each person are enmeshed and other parts are polarized, so they fluctuate between these extremes.

To summarize this section on harmony, family harmony is disrupted by imbalances and burdens, which lead to polarization or enmeshment among family members. Polarized–enmeshed families commonly organize into the same three groups as internal families: exiles, managers, and firefighters. Thus, polarizations and enmeshments constrain family members by forcing them into extreme roles and preventing them from finding and adopting preferred roles. These extremes make it difficult for a family to find and use resources that exist within it for effective leadership.

Leadership

For families to achieve and maintain balance and harmony, they need effective leadership. The qualities of effective family leaders are many and complex. The family therapy literature has focused primarily on the disciplinary aspects of parental leadership, or on helping parents become less enmeshed with their children so that the children can grow up. There are many other aspects of effective leadership that have been given less attention by family therapy. These include the following:

1. Maintaining balance by fairly allocating resources, responsibilities and influence.

2. Monitoring boundaries, which means ensuring that all family members receive the attention, information, and privacy they need to learn and develop, as well as to feel valued and connected. It also means creating an atmosphere in which differences can be expressed, mistakes admitted, problems recognized, and dreams shared—that is, in which issues or feelings are not exiled.

3. Mediating polarizations among members, which requires maintaining the respect and trust of the membership, so that the mediation is considered impartial and wise.

4. Nurturing the development of members. This naturally includes ensuring that their basic material needs are met and that their environment is safe, but also includes making them feel cared for, comforting them when hurt or when family decisions do not go their way, and mentoring them in the sense of encouraging them to find and pursue their personal visions and roles.

5. Relating to systems outside the family. This includes asserting the family's needs and vision, as well as establishing harmonious, sustaining relationships with other systems. It also includes interpreting feedback from other systems to the membership without distortion or delay, and with an eye toward how that feedback reflects possible problems or qualities of the family's structure or values.

6. Personal modeling, which means setting an example for the membership of trying to achieve a balanced and harmonious life and of sacrificing for the larger system while also taking care of oneself. This does not mean hiding the struggles entailed in this achievement, however.

7. Maintaining the family's shared vision. This final aspect of effective leadership is complex enough to require more discussion. Harmonious families generally have an identity—a set of values and goals that is mutually derived and gives each member a sense of connectedness and direction. An effective family leader not only will have a personal vision for his or her life, but also will help the members find their own visions, and will lead family discussions to find commonalities among personal visions that can be assembled into a shared vision.

A Shared Vision

Too often, parents neglect the generative step of establishing a shared family vision, and impose their personal vision on the membership. For example, many parents have powerful dreams for their children—dreams affected by their own disappointments (their personal burdens) or by the extreme values of mainstream U.S. culture, with which they burden their children. In these families, the shared vision becomes rigid and oppressive, without room for difference. In other families, the leaders have little personal vision and little interest in the family's shared vision. Members of these families feel isolated and are guided primarily by self-interest.

What elements are needed for a healthy shared vision? It is my belief that a large part of any shared vision should be to create within the family, and with the systems surrounding it, a sustaining environment. This does not require that the family be perfect in any way, or that it be the biggest, best, most productive, most profitable, or most famous at anything. On the contrary, these striving values can constrain families from becoming sustaining environments. A healthy shared vision may lead one or more family members to become highly productive, famous, or successful, but this will be a by-product of the vision rather than an end in itself. On the other hand, the family may simply be productive enough to survive, and yet can be highly sustaining.

It helps also if the shared vision contains elements of altruism—not just because altruistic goals help humanity, but also because the goal of helping humanity in some way seems to contribute to what is sustaining about sustaining environments. It is often said that people lack meaning in their lives. Working in harmony with others for a cause that transcends personal gain produces meaning. Working exclusively for the gain of the system in which persons are embedded drains meaning from lives, and leads to increasingly narrow, disharmonious vision.

Thus, an effective leader helps the members of the family shape both personal and shared visions that contribute to harmonious, sustaining environments both within and outside the system. To do this, a leader must be able to lead internally with his or her Self, rather than with polarized or extreme parts. When this is the case, the leaders will create a family in which the Selves of the members emerge and feel connected. Another definition of a sustaining environment, then, is a Self-led environment.

Common Leadership Problems

As I have stated repeatedly in this book about human systems in general, families generally have the resources necessary for the kind of visionary, balanced, and harmonizing leadership described here. Those resources are often constrained, however, by a variety of factors that generate problematic leadership styles. These common leadership problems are described below.

Abdicated Leadership

Sometimes the leaders of a family are overburdened. This is one definition of a constraining environment—an environment in which the demands from outside or from within the family are greater than the designated leaders can handle, and the leaders do not delegate responsibilities or do not have anyone to whom they can delegate them. Or a leader may be disabled by injury, by illness, or by extreme parts. When a leader is overburdened or disabled, he or she is likely to abdicate some aspect of leadership. Abdicated leadership creates fear among family members, who will react in a variety of ways, including trying to provoke the leaders back into action by acting out. It also creates a vacuum that others who are ill equipped or inappropriate for the task will try to fill.

Polarized Leadership

In other instances, the leaders of a family are not overburdened, but for a variety of reasons they become polarized with each other. If they cannot contain their polarization within their relationship, polarized leadership results in the problems described in the section on polarization above—coalitions and the need for a distraction. In addition, however, polarized leaders become extreme in opposite directions. For example, one parent may become extremely permissive with the children to counter the other parent's extreme strictness. Each parent would like not to be so extreme, but feels forced to be by the extremeness of the other.

Discredited Leadership

At still other times, a leader may behave in ways that make the members lose trust in or respect for him or her. For example, the leader may not protect the family at a time of crisis or may act selfishly. Or he or she may periodically go on a drinking binge, become abusive, or lie to the membership about important issues. Thereafter, even when the leader displays effective skills, the members do not respond accordingly. To redeem discredited leadership, usually the leader must stop the discrediting behavior, discuss it with the members, apologize, and make reparations where possible. Too often, however, discredited leaders adopt the opposite strategy of denial, pretending that nothing has happened and expecting members to do the same.

Biased Leadership

The final common leadership problem occurs when the leaders favor themselves or one member or group of members over other members. Such biased leadership produces imbalances, which may result in increasing polarization between leadership and the unfavored member or group. To reduce this built-in mechanism for polarization, biased leaders often try to control the family's access to feedback and control the flow of communication within the family ("feedwithin"). In this way, they will either try to keep family members unaware of the imbalances, or justify them as necessary because of some external threat to the family or some larger principle or tradition (e.g., religion or patriarchy).

Handling Feedback and Feedwithin

This brings us to a crucial aspect of leadership. Effective leaders are sensitive to feedback from other systems in the environment, interpret that feedback to the membership without delay or bias, and facilitate the feedwithin process as the family system reacts to the feedback. They trust the ability of the system to find solutions, and react in healthy ways if provided with the necessary information and the ability to communicate freely about it.

Effective leaders also are systems thinkers; that is, they try to interpret feedback with reference to the network of relationships in which their family is embedded or their family's internal structure. For example, when a child fails in school, it is tempting for the parents to think that they just have to push the child harder or help with homework more. But an effective parent will also scan the family system for imbalances, polarizations, or leadership problems that may be constraining, and will similarly assess the child's relationship with peers or with the teacher.

Problematic leadership—whether abdicated, polarized, discredited, or biased—constrains this feedback process. Feedback may not be perceived by abdicated leaders because they are overburdened. Discredited leaders may deny or ignore feedback because it points to their failings. Polarized and biased leaders are likely to overemphasize feedback that supports their positions and to distort or deny other feedback. When feedback regarding the system's performance or the environment's response is ignored, delayed, distorted, denied, or interpreted simplistically, the system is constrained from using its resources to react healthily.

The same thing happens when leaders receive and interpret feedback clearly and without bias, but constrain the family's feedwithin process in response to the feedback. Each type of problematic leadership produces feedwithin problems. Abdicated leaders do not mediate polarizations, allowing them to escalate to destructive proportions. Polarized and biased leaders try to stifle feedwithin from their opponents. Discredited leaders stifle feedwithin that might point to their failings.

Blocked feedwithin escalates polarizations, because members on each side do not receive information regarding the effect of their actions on the rest of the system. They continue their extreme activity, not knowing that they are hurting the larger system or themselves in the long run. In addition, in the absence of direct communication, each side maintains assumptions regarding the motives and nature of the other side that fuel the polarization. I am always amazed at how quickly chronic and disabling polarizations can diminish or disappear, once the opponents speak to one another directly about their real intentions and show other parts of themselves.

Any of the four leadership problems—abdicated, polarized, discredited, or biased leadership—and the accompanying feedback–feedwithin problems can trigger polarizations between the family's leadership and one or more members. That is, one member or a group of members may react to the leadership problem in an extreme way, challenging the family's rules; this challenge then results in an escalating polarization between members and leadership. The leadership problems become lost in the dust created by the challenge and the leaders' attempts to suppress it. In addition, the challengers can become chronic exiles in the system or may be extruded from it.

Finally, leadership problems are rarely as discrete and unitary as I have described them above. Usually an imbalanced and polarized family will exhibit more than one of the four problem styles, because they are contagious. For instance, if a leader abdicates, this change can polarize other leaders, create biases, and lead to discrediting behaviors. One can easily see how any of the four styles can lead to any or all of the other three.

Conclusion

Because this chapter contains an overwhelming number of concepts, I present them here in condensed form in Figure 6.1. This figure lists the

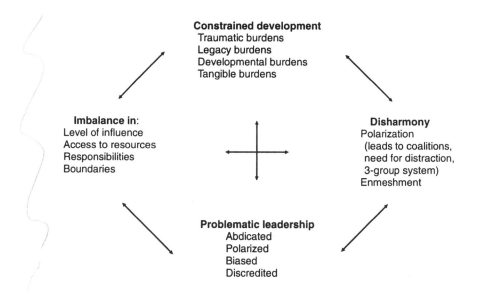

FIGURE 6.1. Summary of problems in the four dimensions of human systems.

common problems within each of the four dimensions, and suggests how problems in each dimension can create problems in each of the others.

In this chapter I have presented the four dimensions in an arbitrary order, suggesting that burdened development creates imbalances, which lead to disharmony, which affects leadership. This is accurate, but it is also accurate that an imbalance can impede leadership, which creates disharmony, resulting in the adoption of a burden. In other words, Figure 6.1 illustrates how a problem in any of the four dimensions can recursively affect each of the others.

To give another example, let's begin with the leadership dimension. After her husband died, a mother of two girls became overwhelmed with depression; she continued going to work, but did little else (abdicated leadership). The elder daughter, 12-year-old Laura, took up the slack, keeping the house clean and making sure her sister was fed and ready for school (imbalanced responsibilities). Laura began binge-eating secretly during this period to deal with her distress. She became harshly critical of her mother and of her 9-year-old sister, Molly (polarization), whose grades dropped precipitously and who began refusing to go to school.

Molly worried about her mother constantly and did not want to leave her side. She developed intense stomach pains, which required enough attention to bring her mother back to awareness for brief periods. The conflicts between her daughters and Molly's somatic symptoms compounded the mother's sense of hopelessness, so she spent more time alone in her room crying. She also formed an alliance with Molly (enmeshment), as they protected each other when Laura attacked either of them (biased leadership), which fueled the existing polarization.

In this example, then, a problem in leadership led to imbalances; these created polarization, enmeshment, and burdens, which further impeded the leadership, and so on. Each family member left this episode with burdens. Each carried grief over the sudden death of the father—grief that remained unresolved because of their individual predicaments. In addition, the mother carried guilt over her abdication and fear because of her collapse. Laura carried the burden of responsibility for the family and, simultaneously, resentment over that responsibility and over being neglected. Molly carried a different kind of responsibility—for the mother's emotional state—and worry over the family's future. These burdens governed the family members' future interactions, as they remained locked in these roles for years.

The dimensions of development, balance, harmony, and leadership become the guidelines I use for helping people find their constraints at any system level. When I meet with a family, for example, I may ask in early sessions about present or past leadership problems; imbalances in resources, responsibilities, or influence; polarizations or enmeshments, or burdens of various kinds. When I work with a person's internal family, I ask about the same things. Or, with either an internal or an external family, I may wait and allow these constraints to emerge out of discussions of problems and solutions. When they do emerge, they become the grist for the therapeutic mill.

CHAPTER 7

Working with Families

In this chapter I present the IFS approach to working with families. At first glance, the prospect of using the IFS model with families may seem dauntingly complex. It is hard enough to keep the parts of one person straight, much less the numerous polarized parts that assemble when the members of a family are convened. Fortunately, however, the IFS model translates into some relatively simple and clear ways of working with and understanding families, which keep the process manageable and enjoyable.

The first of these is inherent in the collaborative relationship the therapist establishes with the family. Since it is a collaboration—a shared responsibility—the therapist does not have to keep track of or change everyone's parts. The therapist does, however, need confidence in his or her Self and awareness of his or her own parts, especially those that may be activated in the course of family therapy.

The Therapist's Role:
Self-Leadership and Parts Awareness

Just as when working with an individual, the IFS family therapist tries to establish a partnership or cotherapy relationship with the Self of each family member. For this to occur, the therapist must be able to lead with his or her Self, sometimes in the face of extreme parts of family members as they activate one another. It is one thing to maintain Self-leadership while working with an individual who has challenging parts, and quite another to do so during scary escalations between wrathful combatants, or while one family member treats another as the therapist's father treated the therapist.

Family therapists have written about the dangers of being inducted into the family's belief system or pattern of interacting. This is a danger because, as in any human system, the parts that govern families are contagious. They will activate the same parts in the therapist.

Possible Induction of Managers

If the therapist has managers that are intolerant of what they consider excessive weakness, neediness, or emotionality, the therapist may collude with the managerial family members to stifle, scorn, or discredit family exiles. For example, a woman complains vehemently to a male therapist that her husband is not available enough. The therapist consistently sides with the husband because he thinks the wife is too needy. Not surprisingly, the therapist's wife has similar complaints.

In addition, because therapists are trying to gain the trust and respect of family members, their approval-seeking parts are often prominent as they interact. With this heightened sensitivity to client feedback, a therapist may be particularly likely to join with the managerial parts of a family. If, for example, a family is holding secrets that the members are afraid will be divulged, that sense of delicateness will be communicated to the therapist. In turn, the therapist's cautious, tentative managers are likely to join the family in tiptoeing around topics that might expose the secrets.

Similarly, the therapist may be intimidated by a family member, because this person could hurt or scare the therapist's own exiles. As a result, the therapist's managers keep him or her at a safe distance from, or placate and ally with, that family member. Or the therapist's fearful parts may be frightened by the extremes of family firefighters. The scared therapist is likely either to join family managers in their coercive attempts to control these firefighters, or to abdicate Self-leadership and allow the firefighters to dominate sessions and the family's life.

Possible Induction of Exiles

Sometimes the therapist identifies with exiled family members, or exiled feelings or issues, to the point where he or she sides with them and exacerbates their polarization with family managers. For example, because the therapist's own exiles are yearning for intimacy or expression, he or she may try immediately to get family members to disclose their most vulnerable feelings. Or the therapist may prematurely take up the cause of a family scapegoat with whom he or she identifies. In these situations, exiled parts of the therapist are upset by the lack of expression in the family or by the attacks on the scapegoat, triggering the therapist's caretaking, angry, moralizing, or rescuing parts. These therapist parts will alienate family managers or set off family firefighters.

In other situations, the therapist's exiles may identify so strongly with the exiled parts of a family member that the therapist is overcome with feeling as the family member gives access to his or her exiles. The family member is likely to sense this and restrict the exile so as to protect the therapist. People are unlikely to raise scary issues or feelings if they do not think the therapist can handle them.

Possible Induction of Firefighters

Sometimes a therapist will react to growing tension in a family session by distracting, or will covertly encourage the distracting activity of a family member who is in the firefighter role. The therapist may automatically make a joke or change the subject, or feel relieved when someone else does these things. In a more extreme example, a therapist with extreme firefighters of his own lived vicariously through his young female client's sexual exploits, asking her to go into great detail. He tacitly encouraged her dangerous trysts and her rebellion against her parents' oppressive managers. Some therapists have such trouble controlling their firefighters that they wind up exploiting clients more overtly, sexually or otherwise.

All of these considerations demonstrate how important it is for the therapist to know his or her own parts and to be aware when they are colluding with or rebelling against family members' extreme parts. The more polarized and delicate the family, the more important this becomes. It is also true, however, that the more a therapist can maintain Self-leadership amid highly polarized family members, the more the therapist's parts trust his or her Self, and the more harmonized the therapist becomes. Thus, doing this kind of work can be very therapeutic for the therapist as well as the family.

Understanding Family Process

In addition to being careful to maintain Self-leadership, the therapist must have a map for understanding complex family interactions and for pacing therapy. Chapter 6 is an attempt to provide such a map. Here, I begin discussing constraints at the family level by exploring family polarizations and enmeshments.

For decades, family therapy theorists have observed that troubled families are characterized by relationships that are either too close or too distant. Below, I first consider the parts patterns of polarized or distant two-person relationships, and then examine the parts patterns of two people who are too close. After that, I expand the focus to include patterns involving more than two people.

Parts Patterns in Polarization between Two People

Since the IFS model views an individual as a tribe of parts and a Self, then a family is a collection of tribes that together form a larger tribal nation of many parts and several Selves. In most polarized families the members have hurt one another, so each individual tribe has exiles that are protected by managers and firefighters. When these tribes conflict, their managers or firefighters are usually the parts that do battle. One person may only show another the explosive Warrior, stoic Computer, impulsive Rebel, apathetic Slouch, rigid Denier, compulsive Caretaker, or any of the myriad other roles into which manager or firefighter parts are forced. These parts try desperately to hide the young, vulnerable exiles that care for the other person, want to be close and loving, and want to play and explore.

As a result of this internecine tribal process, two family members often come to view each other monolithically. Because each only interacts with certain extreme managers or firefighters of the other, each identifies those parts as the whole person, or the person's essence. Thus, many people enter therapy convinced that their children, or spouses, or parents think and feel the extreme things that they demonstrate when in conflict. They only see the protective fortresses of these others, and do not realize that within their walls lie vulnerable, loving, and lovable children.

Manager–Manager Polarizations

Because each member of a polarized pair only sees the other's fortress, each person tries to attack it or break it down with his or her own army of managers, or withdraws defeated within his or her own walls and looks to other people, activities, or substances to ease the loneliness and rejection. Over the years, walls and armies are enlarged. Exiles are more hidden and denied, but also more burdened and easily hurt. Some manager–manager polarizations can be characterized by what family therapists have called "symmetrical escalations" (Bateson & Jackson, 1964), when two tribal armies engage.

In other relationships, a colder war develops between two tribes that have withdrawn behind their respective fortresses; the managers launch occasional missiles at each other from afar. In still other managerial polarizations, we find one person attacking another, who remains entrenched in his or her fortress. In yet others, each person pretends there never was a war and avoids setting foot in the mined territory around the other's fortress.

The characteristic style of any manager–manager polarization depends on which managers of each person step forward to protect the person from the other. We all have preferred protectors; each particular pattern develops from how these preferences fit together. Also, most of us do not depend exclusively on one manager and will shift parts strategically through a conflict. Thus, these managerial patterns cannot always be characterized simply, because they may look different at different points.

Manager–Exile Polarizations

Sometimes a family member's pain or desperation is too much to contain. An exile overwhelms the person's managers and firefighters and stages a coup. Because exiles in polarized families are often chronically neglected and consequently are extremely needy, their desperation is likely to scare other family members. This is especially true when other family members have extreme managers that cannot tolerate vulnerability in themselves or in those around them. Polarizations can then arise between person A's exile and B, the person A has targeted to take care of him or her. The targeted caretaker, B, may fear being smothered or may not know how to relate to hurting exiles. As a result, B reacts with managers, making A feel rejected and even more needy. This triggers a vicious cycle in which each person's parts become increasingly extreme: A feels more hopeless and desperate, and B more trapped and disdainful. This vicious cycle is sometimes broken when A's managers can no longer allow him or her to continue getting hurt. They throw A's exiles back into the fortress, and suddenly distance from or attack B. This shifts the pattern from a manager–exile to a manager–manager polarization.

Manager–Firefighter Polarization

Managers and firefighters are common enemies, even though they both are trying to deal with exiles. Firefighters, in their frantic efforts to douse or dissociate from the fires of feeling, tend to take a person out of control, and managers are often trying to keep the person under tight control. Whenever a person becomes dominated by firefighters, this domination is likely to trigger countering efforts from the person's managers, as well as from managers in the people surrounding the person. Many troubled families are characterized by firefighter–manager polarizations because of this inherent antagonism.

In addition, many troubled families are dominated by extreme manager parts. In these families, even the slightest firefighter activity from one person can trigger extreme controlling reactions in other family members, starting a manager–firefighter vicious cycle. Many of the problems that form the bread and butter of family therapists' practices are characterized, at least at one level, by manager–firefighter polarization. From rebellious acting out to drug or alcohol addiction to under-achievement in school, whenever a firefighter symptom exists, one or more managers are likely to be fueling it.

Whenever extreme or chronic polarization exists in a family, there are also likely to be people who are extremely close. According to the principle of balance in human systems, polarization and enmeshment are complementarily related, as noted in Chapter 6. That is, enmeshment is a common consequence of polarization, and vice versa. The common parts patterns seen in two-person enmeshment are now considered.

Parts Patterns in Enmeshment between Two People

How is enmeshment—especially cross-generational (parent–child) enmeshment—to be understood? Psychodynamic models have pointed to intrapsychic pathology within the parent. Family therapy models have pointed to structural problems within the family. The IFS model suggests that enmeshed parent–child relationships can be maintained by constraints at any number of levels, including the family and intrapsychic, but also including the cultural. Here, however, I focus on the relationship between internal and family patterns in parent–child and other enmeshment.

To return to the principle of balance, if the father of a family has failed to establish an intimate connection with the mother, he may try to find it with his daughter. The father–daughter closeness alienates the mother, who withdraws even further. The same process occurs at the intrapsychic level. If the father has exiled his young, needy parts, so that they get no intimate attention from his Self, then they will desperately seek that attention from outside of him. If his wife has ever reacted to his neediness with critical or cold managers, his exiles may not be allowed to look to her any longer for fear of being hurt again. They look instead to his daughter, because she is available and is safer.

In other words, in this example, the father is trying to get his daughter to nurture the child parts inside him. His exiles are depending on her managers. This reverses the leadership roles, imposing caretaking and protective burdens on the daughter, which constrain her own Self-leadership and exile her own needy parts. She then becomes more likely to form enmeshed relationships with her children when she has them, and parent–child enmeshment is likely to be passed from generation to generation like a chromosome. Thus, in one type of exile–manager enmeshment, one person's exiles feel extremely dependent on and cling to another's managers.

In another form of such enmeshment, a person who has been hurt badly when young often adopts the strategy of trying to enter or become another person. The young parts often believe that if they can get inside the other person, they can get access to that person's power, vitality, confidence, or whatever quality the parts think they lack. They may also believe that if they do not blend with the other person, that person will abandon them. These parts open their boundaries to the other person, and can become confused as to where they stop and the other begins. They try to blend with the strong-appearing managers in the other person—to move, look, and feel as the other does.

Third, as discussed in earlier chapters, many people's exiles carry the burden of worthlessness that was put on them when they were young by abusive or rejecting adults. They become driven to find redemption in the approval of someone who looks, sounds, or acts like the original abuser/redeemer. As a result, the exiles become attached to the managers of the person they perceive as a potential redeemer surrogate. They become desperate for the redeemer's approval, affection, or protection; are willing to do anything to get it; and can only feel good while in that person's presence.

Finally, enmeshment may result from the fear of loss or harm. A person who suddenly lost a parent or child may have exiles that are stuck in time at the period of the loss. He or she will relate to certain other family members out of that fear of an additional loss or abandonment, becoming protectively close to and controlling of those family members.

In some situations, these fears are not the result of being stuck in the past, but are valid in the present. Many families in urban areas of the United States exist in a dangerous, war-zone-like environment. Many of the families we treat at the Institute for Juvenile Research in Chicago live in neighborhoods in which people are killed, raped, or robbed with frightening regularity. Some parents in these families are highly protective of and entangled with their children. Many children are not allowed out of the house except to go to school. This enmeshment may be stifling, but it may be necessary for survival. The children also carry the burden of worry about their parents; for example, they cannot concentrate in school because they want to be home making sure Mom is safe. This protective enmeshment may be necessary within families as well. For example, in a family where the father is violent, the mother and children may band together tightly for mutual protection.

To summarize, there are at least four types of exile–manager enmeshment: (1) A tries to get B to take care of his or her exiles; (2) A tries to get desired qualities from B; (3) A carries the burden of worthlessness and needs B as a redeemer; and (4) A fears loss of or harm to B. For simplicity, I have described these in a linear, A-to-B way. It should be recognized that often the enmeshment is more mutual than this implies and that *B*'s exiles are equally involved.

There are other patterns of two-person enmeshment (e.g., exile–exile, firefighter–firefighter, firefighter–manager), but they all seem to stem from this: The exiles of one or both people feel worthless, frightened, incomplete, neglected, or abandoned. The difference in patterns is related to what parts of *A* are used to try to get things from or protect *B*, and what parts of *B* they are focused on.

Alternating between Enmeshment and Polarization

As mentioned earlier, it is rare to find an intimate relationship that has been always enmeshed or always polarized. Often people alternate between these extremes as one or another set of parts takes control. That is, when person *A*'s neglected exiles take over they will seek intense closeness, while *A*'s protective managers are forced to watch with trepidation from the sidelines. To return to the tribe metaphor, A's starving children break through the barricades of *A*'s fortress and run to *B*'s fortress while *A*'s warriors watch in horror, waiting for *B* to make one false move. At the first sign that these vulnerable children might be hurt by *B*, *A*'s warriors suddenly attack *B* or herd the children back inside *A*'s fortress. Thus, many intimate relationships alternate between periods of intense closeness and extreme conflict or distance.

Family Patterns of Polarization and Enmeshment

Up to this point, I have discussed the common tribal dances of polarization and enmeshment between two people. When we expand the focus to survey a system composed of many family members, we can see how polarizations between two people can coalesce into protective alliances with several family members on each side. We can also see that these coalitions often contain a variety of enmeshed relationships within them.

These family polarizations and coalitions are particularly intense when a family has exiled secrets, issues, or emotions. That is, over the course of a family's life, events or interactions take place that scare or upset key family managers. These events may be related to shameful or frightening past behaviors, such as extramarital affairs, physical or sexual abuse, separations, suicide attempts, or family members' being extruded from the family. These were times when the impulsive firefighters or exiles of one or more family members took over and the consequences were severe. Family managers fear that if certain topics or emotions come up, they could trigger the release of similar dangerous firefighters that they know are still lurking within the family. As a result, they try to prevent those topics or emotions from ever emerging.

In such families, the managers continue to polarize, but the focus of their polarizations will be less threatening issues—ones that are unlikely to activate the exiled feelings or topics. For example, parents may fight over disciplining the kids rather than over why the father is rarely home. Or the family members may focus on how they look and how much they have so as to avoid chronic imbalances. Despite such efforts to contain family exiles, there will be times when these feelings or issues begin to leak through. An argument may begin to escalate beyond the comfortable threshold, or a family member may be stressed to the point where his or her exiles break through the managerial sanctions.

At that point, the family has a need for further distraction. As a result, some family member may be thrust into the role of family firefighter as his or her internal firefighters react to the threatening rise in family tension. The family managers react to counter the acting-out family member, and a new, safer battleground is born. Neither the person in the firefighter role nor those in the manager roles are necessarily aware of the distractive nature of this process. Each person may be reacting automatically, oblivious to the underlying triggers of the reaction, and in great distress over the firefighter–manager polarization in which the parties are embroiled.

I now try to illustrate these ideas with more concrete examples. In many families where a child has the presenting problem, the parents are in managerial roles. Some of these families are so dominated by the parents' managerial parts that firefighters or exiled parts of family members are effectively suppressed for many years. This is true of many families that are dominated by mainstream U.S. cultural values, as I have noted in Chapter 6 and described in detail in Chapter 8. A whole family may be obsessed with appearances and denying of a problem until the problem becomes undeniable. After that, the overt polarizations are those between parents' managers over how best to handle the problem, and those between the parents' managers and the firefighters or exiles of the child who has the problem.

For example, after Judy's boarding school roommate finally told Judy's parents of their daughter's bulimia, they brought her home. While Judy's mother hectored her about what she was doing to them, her father alternated between defending her from the mother and trying to scare Judy about what she was doing to her body. The panicked managers in the parents immediately polarized with Judy's firefighters, who were making her binge. She went from three episodes per week to three per day.

Even prior to this crisis, however, the parents' managers had been polarized with Judy's exiles. Judy often felt neglected by her parents' preoccupation with their careers and with her younger brother's basketball career. She had learned from an early age, however, to hide her sad and lonely feelings, because when she showed them her mother became impatient; she would imply that since Judy had it so much easier than she had had as a child, how could she be unhappy? Her father would change the subject and tell Judy not to dwell on negative thoughts.

Judy's inner managers became parental replicas, exiling her sad and lonely parts and polarizing with her bingeing firefighters, who tried to fill up the seemingly insatiable exiles. She grappled with these parts in secret, fearing that her parents' managerial reactions would only further activate her own managers, thereby increasing her internal polarizations. This was indeed what happened. Now that she was back at home, her own and her parents' managers were taking turns beating up her exiles and firefighters. This made her feel all the more worthless, sad, and lonely, driving her firefighters to work overtime. In addition, the more her parents fought over how to handle her, the guiltier she felt, because she carried the burden of protecting their marriage. This guilt made her managers that much more enraged with her firefighters.

In this example, the parts most directly related to the problem—Judy's bingeing firefighters—were constrained from change not only by having to distract and numb Judy's exiles, but also by the polarization with Judy's and her parents' managers. Judy would have trouble depolarizing her own internal system while her father and mother were constantly activating her parts. If the therapist could first get her parents' managers to back off, then it would be easier for Judy to do the same with her own managers. In addition, if the therapist could get the parents' managers to work together rather than polarize, it would help Judy's worried parts relax.

In other families, the presenting manager–firefighter polarization is seen between the parents, and the children are pulled into roles protecting one or the other of their polarized parents. For example, Barbara's father was a chronic ne'er-do-well who went on frequent drinking binges. Her mother chastised him viciously, often in Barbara's presence. Despite being consumed with resentment, her mother never followed through on threats to throw her father out. Barbara acted as a therapist to her embattled parents, often running from one room to another in a family form of shuttle diplomacy. Barbara was not polarized with either parent over her bulimia. Her mother was worried but tolerant, and her father seemed relatively oblivious. It was as if her parents' battles left little room for other concerns. Barbara's firefighters were activated by her therapist role rather than by polarizations with her parents' managers. She was chronically worried, and felt neglected and alone with her fears.

The point of these examples is that the patterns most evident and accessible in early family sessions are those involving polarizations between family members in managerial roles, or between a family manager and a family firefighter. In some cases, these polarizations are distracting from or are reflective of family exiles—those threatening feelings or issues that the family is afraid to face. In other cases, the presenting polarizations do not seem to be related to family exiles, and problems abate with the resolution of those presenting polarizations.

At this point, I hope that these descriptions of family patterns seem familiar. These are precisely the same patterns I have described for internal families—managers and firefighters trying to contain exiles while polarizing with one another. Not surprisingly, the internal world of a person in each of these family roles is likely to be dominated by the corresponding kind of part. For example, the family taskmaster and peacemaker are probably dominated by managerial parts, the hurt and depressed family members by exiles, and the family rebel and alcoholic by firefighters. Also not surprisingly, the therapist can use precisely the same methods to help family members out of these rigid roles as I have described in earlier chapters for helping parts out of their constricting roles.

Helping Families Change

The rest of this chapter is devoted to describing the practice of IFS family therapy in greater detail. This form of family therapy resembles many other collaborative forms of family therapy, except that (1) the parts language is used frequently; (2) the same ecological sensitivity that is needed in internal work is needed in areas of content for family sessions; and (3) there are two distinct methods of IFS family therapy, which are described after areas of content are explored.

Areas of Content

The first step in working with an external family, just as in working with an internal family, is to join with the system's managers. Family members enter therapy with a wide range of protective feelings. Some feel guilty and are afraid they will be blamed for the problem; others are angry about the problem and the imposition of therapy. All feel some trepidation about trusting the therapist and about what the therapist thinks of them. This fear is accentuated in a case where the family has exiled issues or feelings they fear will be exposed. As a result, family managers are likely to steer therapy toward safer issues and safer polarizations. They will try to define the problem in the safest ways possible—the ways that are least likely to activate exiled issues or feelings.

Reassuring Family Managers

The therapist's first job is to help everyone's protective managers relax as much as possible. The most important way to do that is for the therapist to lead with his or her Self. When the therapist can do this, he or she will be sincerely curious, empathic, accepting, and nurturing, but also confident and direct. These qualities help create a safe environment for the disarming of family members' managers and the emergence of their Selves.

With his or her Self in the lead, the therapist should make respectful contact with each family member, to calm the managers who worry about whether the therapist likes or cares about them. The therapist may encourage these managers to discuss their feelings about being in therapy, and empathize with their natural reluctance to discuss embarrassing issues with a stranger. To reassure managers who worry about what they are getting into, the therapist also emphasizes his or her confidence that together they can solve the problem, and stresses that he or she knows how to proceed. Indeed, the therapist may go into whatever level of detail regarding these methods (the IFS technology, the game plan of therapy) is needed to reduce managerial distrust.

Also in the service of reassuring family managers, the therapist will often initially accept the family members' desire to focus on the problem they present—the one they feel safest with. The discussion of this problem initiates a collective exploration of constraints upon individual family members or upon the family as a whole. Frequently, the IFS therapist begins by exploring the parts of each family member that are constraining them regarding the problem, and then (as described later in this chapter) expands to other levels of constraints—developmental or legacy burdens, problems in the family's current environment, and/or imbalances and polarizations within the family—depending on what is constraining each person's parts.

Introducing Parts Language

Before exploration of the parts connected to the problem can begin, the therapist should introduce the parts language into the session. As described in Chapter 4, this can be done in a natural, almost imperceptible way as each family member describes his or her reactions to the problem. The therapist then repeats what each family member says, but in the parts language. Here is a simple example:

FATHER: When I see that she has binged, I have mixed feelings. I feel sorry for her—that she has to do this to herself—but I also want to slap her and make her see what she's putting us through.

THERAPIST: So one part of you feels sorry for her, but another part gets furious. Is that right?

Because this is how most people talk from time to time, it is rare for anyone to object to statements being rephrased in this way. In fact, many families quickly adopt the parts language and use it as they continue describing their feelings or thoughts.

The parts language in and of itself is a powerful intervention in family sessions. It frees people to disclose more than ordinary language does, because it is easier for a person to acknowledge that a *part* feels or thinks something extreme than to say he or she as a *whole* feels or thinks that thing. It introduces hope, because it is easier for anyone to consider changing a small part than to contemplate changing his or her whole personality. It also implies that each person contains many more resources than are seen in the part of the person most connected to the problem. Finally, it encourages family members to look behind the warring managers or firefighters to see that there are other parts they like or love. Martin Luther King, Jr., had an intuition about this when he said:

> Forgiveness does not mean ignoring what has been done or putting a false label on an evil act. It means, rather, that the evil act no longer remains as a barrier to the relationship. . . . We must realize that the evil deed of the enemy neighbor, the thing that hurts, never quite expresses all that he is. An element of goodness may be found in even our worst enemy.

Thus, simply by using the parts language, a therapist can help family members change the way they see one another. They are not asked to ignore or reframe (put a false label on) the things they have done to hurt one another. They are asked instead to see those hurtful acts as coming from protective parts of one another, and to trust that the other family members are much more than those protective parts.

Tracking Parts Sequences across People

As each family member describes his or her parts that are connected to the problem, the therapist asks questions about how one person's parts affect the others. For example, in response to the therapist's questions, Judy (see above) described a part that criticized her and another part that made her frantic and agitated before she binged. The therapist asked Judy's father how he felt when he saw that frantic part of Judy. He said that he got frustrated and angry because he knew what she was going to do next. He usually tried to contain his frustration, but occasionally he lashed out sarcastically. Judy said that she could tell when his frustrated part was around even when he was silent. She lived in fear of it because it triggered her critic part, which started an internal sequence leading to a binge.

Here, in a few minutes of interaction, Judy and her father outlined a two-person firefighter–manager polarization and the vicious cycle it triggered. Next, the therapist asked Judy's mother how she reacted to her husband's frustrated part and to Judy's frantic part. The mother replied that she also got frustrated with Judy's agitation, but because her husband became so upset, she tended to protect Judy by admonishing him for his outbursts and trying to distract him. She thus described a protective part that could not stand conflict of any kind in her home.

Asking about Change

To continue with the example of Judy's family, at this point each family member identified one or more parts that were activated by their sequences of interaction centering around Judy's bulimia. The therapist continued tracking the impact of each person's parts, and asked each about whether he or she would prefer that a part did not take over. That is, the therapist was asking for descriptions of how their managerial attempts had been ineffective or had even made things worse. With questions such as "So when that frustrated, critical part of you takes over, does it help things?", the therapist helped each family member acknowledge that they would prefer to respond to one another differently.

THERAPIST: (*to father*) What do you say to yourself when you know she's binged?

FATHER: I feel disgusted and like I've got to stop her.

THERAPIST: Judy says that when that frustrated part of you takes over, it makes her self-critical and more likely to binge. Were you aware that this part of you had that impact?

FATHER: She's told me, and I can tell that I make her more frantic and disgusted with herself, but I can't seem to stop myself. I can't stand to see her do this to herself. It's so hard to sit by and feel powerless.

THERAPIST: Do you think it would be more helpful to Judy if you could stay your Self with her, so she knew you still cared about her?

FATHER: Probably. I do love her, but I can see how it would be hard for her to always know that. My love gets covered up by this frustration.

I could try to be more patient, but this situation is so painful for me that I'm sure I'll keep getting frustrated.

THERAPIST: So you would like to keep that frustrated part from interfering in your relationship with Judy, but you don't know how to do that. Is that right?

FATHER: Yes, that's right.

Such questions also bring a shared vision into the family—that is, a shared image of the preferred future. As discussed in Chapter 6, shared vision is an essential quality of good leadership and of healthy human systems. Such vision is easily obscured by polarized parts. As polarizations dissipate and parts step aside, family members can describe how they would prefer to relate; as they do so, their Selves can create the vision and the accompanying hope that were previously missing.

THERAPIST: If you and Judy could keep your parts from interfering in your relationship, what might it look like?

FATHER: I want to be able to talk with Judy about her life. Not that she has to tell me everything she does or talk to me all the time, but I'd like to get to know her again and be able to give her some advice from time to time.

Family members are not always so willing to implicate their own parts in problems. At least one member may insist that another person's parts, not his or her own, need to change. When that is the case, the therapist does not need to convince the person that his or her parts are involved in the problem. Instead, the person will usually agree that his or her attempts to change the other person's parts have failed or backfired. Consequently they will agree to a temporary moratorium on trying to change the other's personality, as long as the person believes that the therapist is helping the other to do this. With that agreement in place, each person may be willing to work on the parts of him or her that are upset by the problem.

To summarize the process up to this point, the therapist asks all family members for their vision of how they would like things to be, asks what parts of them get in the way of that, and asks whether they are interested in changing those constraining parts.

Reassuring Managers in Regard to Proposed Change

Once family members have acknowledged that they wish to change their relationship with parts of them, the therapist lets them know that he or she can help them do that, and asks whether they are interested in his or her help. At that point the concerns of one or more persons' managers are likely to be voiced, and the therapist simply addresses each concern sincerely and in a straightforward manner.

THERAPIST: If you are interested, I can help you with that frustrated part. It sounds like it's triggered by a part that cares a great deal about Judy and is extremely pained to see her suffer.

FATHER: That is true. If I didn't care, I wouldn't get so frustrated.

THERAPIST: When you are ready, I can help you with that caring part too—not so that you stop caring, but so that it isn't intolerably painful. Would you be interested in working with these parts of you?

FATHER: I'll do anything to help Judy, but I don't think I'm the only problem.

THERAPIST: I agree. We've already talked about parts of Judy and of Mrs. R that are involved, and I'll be asking each of them if they are willing to work on their parts. The goal is for everyone in the family to work together to keep their parts from interfering, so you can better show the caring you have for each other.

FATHER: Are you saying that this part of me is causing Judy to be bulimic?

THERAPIST: No, not at all. We're just trying to create the best environment possible for Judy to work with the parts of her that are involved in her bulimia. While her parts are constantly activated by your Frustrated Guy, it's harder for her. If you can stay your Self with her, it makes her work easier.

FATHER: I guess that makes sense. But before I try this, I want to know what I'm agreeing to do. What do you mean by helping me work with my part?

At this point, the father's (as well as the mother's and Judy's) managers were wondering what they were getting into. They were worrying about what they might be asked to do in front of the others and whether this process was safe. In her statements about the process, the therapist tried to calm everyone's managers.

THERAPIST: There are a lot of different ways to do that, and we would find the one you are most comfortable with. For example, I could have you focus on this Frustrated Guy during the week, and when you feel or hear him, have you just ask him to step back. So that way involves simply being more aware and changing some thought patterns. Or I could ask you to see the part and have you work with it through imagery. Or we could act as if I was speaking directly to the part in a kind of role play.

What's important to know is that because there are many different ways, you cannot fail at this. We will find a comfortable way that works for you. Also, I know how to do this safely, and you will be in total control of the pace and the content. I never go farther or faster than you are comfortable with. When you are ready, you will be able to choose whether you want privacy or you are okay having Judy and Mrs. R watch. At any point, I can ask them to leave the room. We all have things we would prefer to work on in private, and we want each of you to feel as safe as possible. Sometimes there are advantages to having family members watch—for example, they may feel more empathy for what you struggle with—but I want everyone to feel as safe as possible.

A therapist's confident demeanor; his or her nonblaming, optimistic, multiplicity-oriented perspective; and reassurances regarding safety and control all serve to deactivate managers in each family member simultaneously. The therapist is bringing Self-leadership into a system that has had little access to such leadership.

At this point, the therapist may have conversations similar to the one above with the other family members regarding the way their parts interfere and their willingness to try to change that. As each family member sees that the others are acknowledging some role in the problem and some motivation to do their part to help, each member's managers are further reassured. As the atmosphere in the session feels safer and managers relax, family members will begin to show more Self-leadership in the way they respond to one another.

Selecting the Level of Focus

At this point, the therapist and family have many choices in the direction they might proceed. The direction they select will depend on which system level (internal systems, certain family relationships, nuclear family, extended family, work, school, community, or culture) they think would be the best one on which to begin to focus, and what would be the best way to address the constraints at that level. The therapist can present the options to the family and make the decision a collaborative one.

THERAPIST: Now that we have an idea of some of the parts of each of you that are stuck to this problem, we need to find out what is keeping these parts in their extreme roles. These constraints may exist at any number of levels. We have already talked a little about the internal level—about how your parts operate inside you—but there are things in your relationships with each other and in your lives outside the family that will also affect your parts. For example, Mr. R, your Frustrated Guy is obviously activated by Judy's frantic part. But we could also talk about how your job affects that frustrated part. Or how the balance of responsibilities in the house affects Mrs. R's protective part. Or how Judy's interactions with peers affect her critical part. I need to know from all of you where you think the biggest constraints exist.

MOTHER: Well, I know that Paul's job frustrates him. There are times where he comes home from work with a real chip on his shoulder. I don't blame him for it because he's under a lot of pressure. I just try to stay out of his way at those times.

In this way, the therapist can expand the focus of therapy from the level of internal parts to any level that seems fruitful, and can go back to the parts again whenever this is appropriate. The family members can discuss external constraints and what to do about them, while simultaneously discussing how their parts react to these external constraints.

Shifting Levels

At this point, I hope the reader is getting a picture of IFS family therapy as a highly collaborative and fluid process. The focus of therapy will shift from the internal to the external and back again without any disruption, because the world is viewed as one huge system containing systems at several levels. In addition, changes at the external level of family relationships can create corresponding changes within family members, and vice versa. Therefore, a therapist can focus at either level and know that he or she is affecting the other level.

One reason for this is the principle of "parallelism." This principle states that person A will often relate to person B in a way that parallels A's relationship with the parts of A that resemble B. For example, when Mrs. R (Judy's mother) was sad, Mr. R often treated her the same way he treated his own sad exiles. He became agitated and gave her advice in an impatient, critical voice. The principle of parallelism would suggest that if Mr. R became able to nurture his exiles, this could translate into his being more nurturing toward his wife's exiles, even if the issue of his lack of nurturance was never directly addressed. It would also suggest the reverse: If he could maintain Self-leadership with his wife when she was sad, he would be better able to care for his exiles.

Thus, the IFS therapist is free to work at whatever level seems most effective and ecologically sensitive, secure in the knowledge that other levels are shifting simultaneously. In my work with some families and couples, we never dealt directly with anyone's internal system because it did not seem comfortable or necessary. I still used the parts language and often asked family members to move parts that were interfering, but I never used in-sight or direct access, because it seemed that the work at the external level was resolving the problems and creating harmony. With other families, we worked primarily at the internal level of each family member, and family relationships changed dramatically without ever being directly addressed.

Asking about Burdens

Up to now in this chapter, I have focused mainly on how to help family members depolarize, maintain Self-leadership, and work with their parts. Although the content of this work will often involve the constraining effects of the different parts of family members that are involved with the problem, as discussed above, other important areas of content may not emerge through those discussions. These areas may not emerge because they are connected to exiled issues or feelings that family managers are afraid to address.

Chapter 6 has described how family burdens create family imbalances, which in turn create family polarizations and leadership problems. So far, this chapter has suggested that the initial focus of therapy should be on family polarization and leadership in relation to the problem. This is a convenient starting point because it often feels safest to family managers. Since burdens and imbalances are interrelated with polarizations and leadership problems, the initial focus on the latter will often lead to the former. When it does not, however, and when a family appears significantly constrained by developmental, legacy, or tangible burdens or by chronic imbalances, the therapist should ask questions designed to invite the family to explore those areas of content as well, even those that are exiled.

Family burdens are often less threatening to discuss than imbalances. For this reason, the therapist may want to start with questions about burdens, which can then lead to questions about imbalances. For example, it is often safer for members of a family to discuss whether they carry the burden of patriarchy from the parents' families of origin or their cultural backgrounds than it is to discuss how the father currently has more influence, more resources, and fewer household responsibilities than the mother. Yet discussing the burden of patriarchy can flow smoothly into a conversation regarding whether that burden has created current family imbalances. If the imbalances are viewed as related to burdens, they carry less blame, and consequently may become less polarizing.

Family Developmental Burdens. A family is often constrained by burdens resulting from events in the family's distant or recent history, yet these events do not emerge as issues in the therapy. When a family does not spontaneously report powerful events, it may indicate that the events are exiled from family discussion or awareness. Often the burdens from these events lurk like ghosts within family sessions, exerting a powerful, unseen influence. The therapist may sense that something does not fit—that there seems to be a missing piece in the puzzle.

Once family managers begin releasing their grip on family conversations, the therapist may want to ask about burden-generating events. These may include unmourned deaths, abusive episodes, disabling illnesses, marital separations, drug or alcohol binges, or the like; alternatively, they may be events that seem innocuous to the therapist but have special meaning to family members. Often, once such a burdening event is revealed and discussed, it seems as if the family is frozen in time around the event in much the same way that internal parts become stuck in the past.

In some cases, a burdening event triggered the problem that the family now presents. Thus, the therapist may ask about the onset and history of the problem, and about how its timing corresponds to difficult or traumatic periods in the family's life. In addition, burdening events can be traced backward from the way their burdens manifest in present. That is, as extreme parts emerge in family sessions, the therapist can ask about the origin of the parts' beliefs or feelings.

THERAPIST: Mrs. R seems to have a tremendous fear of losing Judy. Has anything happened in the family's life that might have given her this burden of fear?

FATHER: I don't know if this is related, but we had a miscarriage and a stillbirth before we had Judy. It was hard on both of us, but we just pressed on and put it all behind us once Judy arrived. I haven't thought much about that since, but maybe it's had an unconscious impact on us.

The therapist then led a discussion of the impact of those events and burdens on the family's life. In addition, the therapist had Mr. and Mrs. R go inside and ask if any parts held the feelings about those events. Through internal and external conversation, the family members decided what they needed to do to release the burdens accrued from the events. Mr. and Mrs. R discussed their interactions during and after those events, and Mr. R apologized for not being more available during those periods to console his wife. He said that his way of handling grief was to forget about it, so he couldn't stand to be around her while she cried. Mrs. R expressed her resentment at being abandoned during that terrible period; described her desperation to have a child; and relived her terror of losing Judy to her childhood asthma, even though it was mild. During this disclosure, she wept openly, and Mr. R was able to hold her in a way he never could before. In addition, both parents worked with their burdened parts in each other's presence.

Cultural and Legacy Burdens. In the same way that the therapist identifies developmental burdens from the way those burdens manifested in sessions, the therapist can also ask about cultural and legacy burdens—that is, burdens accrued from an intergenerational transfer process, which is discussed in Chapter 8.

THERAPIST: (*to father*) Where did you get this belief that men are entitled to more free time at home?

FATHER: Well, that was the way it was in my family, and I guess I picked it up from the way my parents operated.

Or the therapist can begin by asking parents to describe their respective families or ethnic cultures, to discuss the burdens they carried, and then to discuss how many of those burdens are still with the family and how they are manifested in the family.

FATHER: My father could never give me a break. No matter how well I did in school, he could never bring himself to compliment me. He always found a way to let me know it was not good enough.

THERAPIST: So he carried the burden of perfectionism. Judy, do you think your father has a part that inherited this burden?

JUDY: I'll say! Maybe not in the same way exactly, because Dad does compliment me sometimes. But I always have the feeling around him that I'm not quite good enough, like I'm disappointing him—even when he compliments me.

THERAPIST: And do you think you have a part that inherited this perfectionism from him?

JUDY: Well, I don't criticize anyone but my parents and myself. But, yeah, I guess I'm always judging people in negative ways, even if I don't say anything to people about it. But I'm harder on myself than anyone else.

THERAPIST: (*to all family members*) How do you think this burden of perfectionism that you inherited from Mr. R's family has affected your family?

The family members then discussed further who carried the burden, how they each reacted to it, and how they could work together to help one another release it. They also speculated on where the father's family of origin first picked it up. They reviewed the hardships and rejections that Judy's great-grandparents had endured as Jewish immigrants at the turn of the century, as well as the discrimination her grandparents had endured during World War II.

In addition, a family inherits some values or emotions from its culture that are not burdensome per se, but become burdensome when they do not fit with the family's current circumstances. The therapist can ask about the values or structure of the parents' families of origin, how similar or different the values or structure of the present family is, and how well those similarities or differences fit the family members' lives now.

Finally, also as described in Chapter 8, there are many aspects of mainstream U.S. culture that create burdens; it is often useful to help family members discuss which of these cultural burdens they carry and whether they want to continue carrying them. Such burdens include competitive and materialistic striving, isolating appearances and self-consciousness, self-reliance, patriarchy, and racism.

Tangible Burdens. Tangible burdens, as discussed in Chapter 6, are the constraints imposed on the family by their current circumstances. In this sense, tangible burdens are different from developmental, legacy, and cultural burdens, in that their constraining effect is not (or is only to a limited extent) the result of extreme ideas or feelings. Tangible burdens may include stressful jobs, the effects of poverty and of racial or sexual discrimination, and the dangers of the neighborhood. They may also include the special needs of disabled or elderly family members, or any other circumstances that drain a family's leadership and resources. Questions about tangible burdens can include what they are, what their impact on the family is, whose parts are the most affected by them, and how the family members can work together to diminish their impact.

Asking about Imbalances

Burdens create imbalances. As the reader will recall from Chapter 6, families can become imbalanced in four different areas: degree of influence, access to resources, level of responsibilities, and boundaries. Once the atmosphere of therapy feels safe and trusting enough for the family members to handle exiled issues and feelings, the therapist can ask questions regarding the balance in key family relationships in these areas. Here are some examples:

- How are key decisions made in the family? How does this work? (That is, who has input? Who has final say?)
- Who has access to the most and the least leisure time, money, attention, friends, and so forth? How is that decided in each case?
- Who has the most and the least responsibility in the family? How is that decided?
- Who is closest to whom? Who is most distant? Who is most protective of whom? How possible is it for two family members to engage in conflict without the interruption of a third?

Each of these questions can be followed by a series of related questions designed to assess the impact of any imbalances found in those areas:

- Who has parts that are afraid to discuss the imbalance? What are they afraid might happen?
- How does that imbalance affect parts of each of you?
- What arrangement might feel better?
- What keeps you from having it that better way? Whose parts would object?
- What are you afraid would happen if things were more balanced?
- How do you think this imbalance affects the parts of each of you that are stuck to the problem?

Frequently these questions lead to exiled issues, and consequently they are frightening to family managers. If the family members express (either overtly or covertly) strong fear about discussing an imbalance, the therapist may want to lead a discussion of those fears first. Family members will often become less afraid as they examine these fears openly, with their Selves in the lead.

These questions about family imbalances, as well as those about burdens, not only elicit useful information; they are also powerful interventions in and of themselves. They tend to elicit Self-leadership within the family. This is because the questions require what I call a "metaperspective"—an ability to step above the fray and look down at the family's predicament. It is a person's Self, more than any part, that has this metaperspective, and so family members' Selves are often elicited by the questions. When the family members can communicate from this Self-led metaperspective, they can view their predicament with more compassion and can see solutions that were obscured by the tunnel vision of their parts.

Methods of Family Therapy

Up to this point, I have focused primarily on the content of IFS family sessions. The methods presented above have included using the parts language and asking questions designed to elicit burdens or imbalances. Now I focus on two methods that are the foundation of IFS family therapy: maintaining Self-leadership and working with one person's parts.

Maintaining Self-Leadership: The Parts Detector

During discussions of constraints surrounding the problem, it is expected that parts of family members will overtake them as they talk. When the therapist detects this, he or she can stop the action, ask each family member to see whether a part has taken over, and ask that part to step back and trust his or her Self to lead. Thus, the therapist develops a "parts detector"—a sense of when people are and are not leading with their Selves—and uses it to help family members maintain Self-leadership as they interact.

Negotiating a Truce between Parts. This way of maintaining Self-leadership is one of the two primary methods of IFS family therapy. For example, if the family wants to work on a particular relationship, the therapist organizes the two people involved to face each other and begin talking about their issues. As their parts pop up and begin to escalate, the therapist stops them; both persons are asked to go inside and find out what their parts are upset about. Next, they are asked to come back and speak for their parts rather than having the parts take over. In this way, both persons gain trust in their Selves, because they see that things go better when the Selves lead. In addition, the issues between them are often resolved quickly, because the rigidity of their parts was what was maintaining the issues. Now they feel heard, even empathized with, and suddenly solutions are more available.

FATHER: (*to Judy*) The only time you are decent to me is when you want something. You're spending all your life in your room doing God knows what, and I'm just supposed to go along with this!

JUDY: And all you want is to control me. I don't talk to you because I don't really like you . . .

THERAPIST: (*cutting Judy off*) Okay, stop the music for a second. I'd like each of you to go inside and talk to your parts about what they want and why they are taking over. Let me know when your Self is back.

JUDY: (*after a long silence*) Okay, I'm back.

THERAPIST: Can you tell your father what was going on?

JUDY: My angry part gets going whenever you complain about the time I spend in my room. I feel bad about that too, but when I feel so ashamed of how I look, I need to withdraw. And when you get on me about it, I feel worse about myself. There's another, younger part that feels like you see me as a failure. Whenever you comment on my problems, that part feels horrible.

FATHER: I'm sorry ... I let my Frustrated Guy go again. He's just so worried about you and desperate to get you past this. When you hole up in your room, the house feels empty and I know you're up there suffering, so I can't feel like things are okay. I also feel like I'm failing as a father.

Here Judy and her father were negotiating a truce between their respective managers. In other words, they were beginning to depolarize a two-person, manager–manager polarization. His manager was controlling and hers was withdrawing. With their Selves in the lead, they could speak for some of the other parts that these managers were protecting, and thereby could let each other peek behind the managerial walls. As they continued and it felt safer, they could gradually let these other, more vulnerable parts out and could enjoy each other again.

Monitoring the Effects of Change. As this warming of Judy's relationship with her father continued, her mother's parts reacted. The mother's and Judy's relationship had been enmeshed; each had feared the loss of the other. Therefore, parts of both were threatened by this change. With this and every change, therefore, the therapist asked how the parts of other family members were reacting to it.

THERAPIST: Mrs. R, how would it be for you if Judy and Mr. R got closer?

MOTHER: I think it would be great. It would be a big relief because I could get out of the middle, and I think it would be healthy for both of them.

THERAPIST: I'm glad you feel that way. If I were you, however, I would also have some parts that feared losing the closeness I had with Judy. You two have been close for a long time, and this might mean a change in that.

MOTHER: (*defensively*) Are you saying that I want them to be distant so I can hold on to Judy?

THERAPIST: No, not at all. Just that there might be a small part of you that is insecure about this change and might need some reassurance. Any change in a family is disconcerting to parts of family members. Would you mind going inside for a second, just to see if everybody is okay about this change?

MOTHER: (*after a pause*) Well, there is one part of me that is having trouble in general with Judy getting older and growing up. It's the part of me that so enjoyed having a little girl and misses that little girl. I think that's natural, though. Every mother experiences that.

THERAPIST: It's perfectly natural. I have that part, and I suspect Mr. R has a part like that too. Judy may also have a part that is afraid to get older and grow up and misses being a little girl. Sometimes there are ways to help those parts feel better when you hear more about what they fear and what you could do for them.

In addition to checking with other family members about a pending change, it is also important to ask about other parts of those involved in the change.

THERAPIST: Judy, are there any parts of you that are afraid to get along better with your dad?

JUDY: Well, yeah, I'm afraid it won't last. I'll let him get close and then he'll be mean again.

THERAPIST: Is there also a part that worries about your mother's reaction?

JUDY: Yeah, there's a part that worries about her all the time—not just about this, but about everything with her. I can't stand it when she's upset, and I'm not sure if she'll be okay with this.

To summarize, during this process a therapist is doing several things. First, he or she tries to maintain Self-leadership within the family by asking family members to find parts as they emerge and to speak for their parts rather than through them. Second, the therapist asks family members to talk, with their Selves in the lead, to one another about their issues. Third, as the family's Self-leadership begins to produce change, the therapist asks family members about the reaction of their parts to the pending change, and helps them deal with those parts and decide on the best pace for change.

Working with One Person's Parts

In addition to this process, however, there will be times where it is important to work with the parts of one or another family member more directly. In Judy's family, for example, at one point or another the therapist might ask Judy to work with her withdrawing manager or the hurt parts it protected, or might ask the father to work with his Frustrated Guy, or might ask the mother to work with those of her parts that feared losing Judy.

Observation by Family Members versus Work in Private. This work with one family member's parts can happen in a number of different ways, depending on what feels most comfortable to the person and family. Where it feels safe to the family member doing the work, it can be helpful to have him or her work in the presence of other family members. The observing family members often feel a profound empathy for the one doing the work, and understand that person in a different way. For example, Judy and her mother watched Mr. R struggle with his Frustrated Guy. They saw that this part was critical and controlling not only with them, but even more so with Mr. R himself. They heard him describe how the Guy was stuck in the past at age 12, when his father was slowly dying of cancer and he had to sit by, powerless to help him. As a result, they could understand and experience his desperation in a new way, and felt united with his Self in an effort to release the Frustrated Guy from desperation. In addition, Mr. R felt a kind of acceptance from his wife and daughter that he had never before experienced, because they seemed so nurturantly responsive to this vulnerability.

Although having other family members observe can result in these salubrious consequences, it will often feel risky to the person doing the work. That person is being asked to be vulnerable in front of people who have hurt him or her in the past and might do so again. Even when the work seems successful in the session, the person's managers are likely to be on red alert afterward because he or she has been so vulnerable, and the person may lash out at the observers for the slightest sign that they are not accepting. The therapist is well advised to warn the family that a period of protectiveness often follows such a session.

In addition, even when a family seems to contain a high degree of Self-leadership, it is hard to predict what parts of the observers will be activated as they observe. For example, if as Mrs. R watched, she had been overcome by the part of her that felt so angry at and hurt by the Frustrated Guy in Mr. R, she would have received a distorted view of the work he did and might have attacked him for it. This would make Mr. R more reluctant to disclose and more protective. When a family member does work in front of others, then, the therapist should save time to ask the others about parts of them that were activated while they observed. The therapist should help them separate from those parts so that they can respond from their Selves, and should predict trouble if they cannot separate.

Thus, because this is a delicate process it is important to give all family members complete freedom of choice in whether or not they are observed by the others. When the therapist fears that a person may feel uncomfortable asking for privacy, the therapist should insist they begin in private. The therapist then either asks the other family members to wait in the waiting room or schedules an individual appointment with the person.

After a family member has worked in private with his or her parts, family empathy and understanding can be generated if the person is willing to tell the other family members something about what happened. Even this level of disclosure may be threatening or dangerous for the person, and, again, he or she is free to choose total confidentiality regarding the parts work. If the person decides to disclose, he or she can discuss with the therapist before talking to the family what feels safe to reveal, so that nothing is disclosed that might later be regretted.

Other Considerations. There is a rule that can help family members feel safer in exposing their parts to one another. The rule is that no one can comment on another person's parts outside the sessions. Each person can, however, speak about his or her own parts, and I often encourage this. This rule is designed to prevent family members from exploiting sensitive information by telling one another to get rid of or bring forward parts they have learned about in the sessions. Thus, statements such as "I know you've got a little boy in there, so get that angry part out of my face and let me talk to him," are not allowed. On the other hand, such statements as "A part of me feels scared by your anger, and I need a second to calm it down," are encouraged.

This rule is primarily important and enforced while the family shows little Self-leadership. While this is the case, it is usually A's parts (not A's Self) making comments about B's parts. The "get that angry part out of my face" statement above is likely to be delivered by a part that is insisting that the other person change. When a part of A tries to change a part of B, it usually backfires, making B's part more extreme and polarized with the part of A. Once Self-leadership is more clearly evident in the family, it is possible to lift the rule, because A's Self can help B with his or her parts.

With many family cases, each family member will have at least one session in which the focus is on his or her parts. Sometimes the therapist will suspend the family sessions temporarily and work intensively with one family member's parts for a series of sessions. In other situations, the therapist will try to maintain a balance and have family members work on their parts in sequence; in the R family's case, for example, the focus could have alternated among Judy, her mother, and her father in the sessions. Whenever possible, decisions regarding who to work with and when are made in collaboration with the family during discussions of their constraints.

These discussions should include how family members would feel if one person did more internal work than another. When the therapist works with one family member's parts and not another's, the danger exists that the person doing the work will believe, or the others will believe, that he or she is the most disturbed, has the biggest problem, or, on the other hand, is the therapist's favorite. To avoid that perception, the therapist should offer to work with each family member, and should make it clear that the one doing the most parts work is often the one most courageous and motivated to help the problem change, or perhaps the one most curious about his or her inner life.

The Self-Confidence Technique. When Bowen (1978; Kerr & Bowen, 1978) worked with an individual, he frequently sent him or her on a "family-of-origin voyage." That is, he had the person meet with family members between sessions where they would strive to maintain some degree of self-differentiation and to avoid induction into the family's preferred interaction patterns. The IFS therapist can work with a person in a similar way. For example, Mrs. R felt perpetually hurt by her own mother's comments criticizing her parenting skills and blaming her for Judy's problems. While her family watched, the therapist used an in-sight method called the "Self-confidence technique" to help Mrs. R's parts trust her Self to deal with her mother.

THERAPIST: In your mind, put your mother in a room by herself, and you stay outside the room with your parts. In a minute I'll ask you to go into the room as your Self, with your parts waiting safely outside. First, though, talk with your parts about what they want you to say to your mother when you go in, and find out who is afraid to let you go in without them.

MRS. R: (*after a pause*) Okay. Initially there was an argument about what to say to her, but they compromised. Now there's an angry part that won't let me go in by myself.

THERAPIST: Do you think you can get it to trust you for just a little while?

MRS. R: (*after a long pause*) I told it that I understood its fears, but that I knew I could handle her if I didn't have to worry about those young parts getting hurt. I asked it to look after them while I was in the room.

Mrs. R then entered the room as her Self and asked her mother why she was so critical of her. After first responding caustically, her mother softened and said that she was resentful of Mrs. R because she was always so close to her father. Mrs. R was surprised to hear this and told her mother so, but it helped her make sense of a lot of things in their relationship. After finishing this inner conversation, Mrs. R left the room and asked her parts how they thought she did as their spokesperson. They seemed very pleased and amazed that she could be so strong, although one part insisted that she could never do that in reality. She asked her parts to let her do this *in vivo*, and they said they would try. The next week she asked her mother to lunch, and indeed had a very similar conversation with her. Although her mother did not spontaneously acknowledge being jealous of Mrs. R's relationship with her father, the mother conceded when Mrs. R asked about this that she did feel neglected by him at times and felt left out of the father–daughter relationship.

This is called the Self-confidence technique because it is designed to foster trust in the Self's leadership. After watching her Self handle things so well with her mother, Mrs. R's parts had more confidence in her Self's leadership in other arenas of internal and external life. They felt less need to protect her and were more trusting that she could protect them. This technique can be used in a wide variety of contexts and for a variety of purposes. With Mrs. R it was used in a family therapy context, but it is also used extensively in individual or couples therapy. The stimulus for the technique can be anything—a relationship with a living or dead person, or a situation that is anticipated or that happened in the past. The person does not have to follow up the internal Self-confidence work with comparable external work, because the internal work alone is often very powerful.

Conclusion

This chapter is complex because there are a large number of ways to use the IFS model with families. Therapists should remember that they can start with any of these methods or content areas and easily shift to another, because they are all interrelated; they are all tied to the parts of each of the family members. Therapists should also remember that they do not have to use this form of family therapy precisely as described here. Many of the ideas and methods can be easily grafted from the IFS model onto the form of family therapy that a reader is more comfortable with.

CHAPTER 8

Applying the Model at the Cultural and Societal Levels

Two souls, alas, do dwell within his breast; the one is ever parting from the other.

–Goethe, Faust, *Part I*

Faust complained that he had two souls in his breast. I have a whole squabbling crowd. It goes on as in a republic.

–Bismarck

Thus far in this book, the IFS principles have been applied to individuals and to families. The cultures and the society in which families and individuals develop and live have a tremendous impact on them. This chapter discusses aspects of middle-class mainstream U.S. culture and contrasts those with generalizations about ethnic cultures and the families they produce. Although at times this discussion may seem far removed from the intrapsychic framework presented in Chapter 2, it is not. To fully understand the extremes of an internal system, one must understand the cultural and societal context in which these extremes develop and are maintained.

I then introduce three kinds of families: "hyper-Americanized," "transitional," and "tradition-based." Each of these types contains imbalances, polarizations, and leadership problems, but for different reasons relating to their different cultural development and their current cultural circumstances.

The Parts and Self of a Society

Can we conceive of a society in the same way we conceive of an individual or a family? To apply the IFS principles to a society, we have to see it as a large human organism composed of smaller groups (parts) that interact. If we target U.S. society as a whole, we can view it as composed of any number of different kinds of groups, depending on our lens. That is, if we use a political lens, we might see liberals, conservatives, feminists, religious fundamentalists, and so forth. If we use a socioeconomic lens, we might see the poor, the working class, the middle class, the upper class, and the various subgroups comprising these classes.

In this chapter, however, I use primarily the lens of ethnicity. Through ethnicity, we see U.S. society as dominated by a set of "American" cultural values, conveyed through the mass media and lived by a minority of the population. Within this society also exist a large number of different cultures, with value systems differing from from that of the dominant or mainstream culture. Each ethnic group has a different relationship with the mainstream group and with other ethnic groups. Some groups are polarized with the mainstream and become exiles, and others are embraced and elevated in stature. Several groups are polarized with one another. If we were to imagine U.S. society as a person, that person would be dominated by a few parts (most likely striving, evaluating, and asserting parts); other parts would be exiled by the managerial coalition because they were seen as lazy or dangerous; and still others would be accepted and employed because they were viewed as industrious and competent.

What is the counterpart to the Self within a society? Ideally, it is the government, which, if it is leading effectively, will demonstrate the same qualities I have described for effective family leaders in Chapter 6. Unfortunately, in the United States the government exhibits each of the four types of problematic leadership also described in that chapter. Too often our political leaders are biased, polarized, discredited, and abdicating. Of these four, the most problematic is the built-in bias whereby only people from the dominant group can afford to become political leaders, and these can only do so with the help of others in the dominant group. Biased leadership, then, maintains or exacerbates the imbalances and polarizations among the groups in U.S. society. The threat produced by the resulting polarizations further biases leadership against the exiled groups.

Cultural Burdens

To continue the analogy to a person, all the parts of a society (the component cultural groups) carry burdens accrued from the traumas of their histories. For example, the early American settlers (the British and other Europeans), whose values have evolved into those of what I am calling the dominant, managerial coalition, were generally persecuted or troubled in their own countries and faced what they considered a very hostile and dangerous environment in the New World.

In addition, they carried a legacy burden of racism. European racism was in existence long before the settlers arrived, as exemplified by the "doctrine of discovery." This was the policy used by the New World explorers to justify the brutal conquest and enslavement of indigenous peoples. In essence, it was a declaration of war against all non-Christians throughout the world; it emanated from decrees issued by Pope Nicholas V in 1452, 40 years before Columbus's big "discovery." In these decrees, non-Christians were portrayed as enemies of Catholicism, and as such were considered less than human. Christian European nations were encouraged to vanquish the pagans—to take all their possessions and property, and to put them into perpetual slavery (Newcomb, 1992).

These burdens of fear, anger, and racism account for the generally barbaric and exploitive ways in which European invaders treated Native Americans, and, later, for their embracing the inhuman institution of slavery for 300 years. The hardships encountered by the European settlers added fear and pain to their racist burdens. They became dominated by aggressive, individualistic, striving, and righteous parts that had very little compassion for those different from or in competition with them. Centuries later, mainstream U.S. culture remains burdened by this same aggressive, individualistic, striving, righteous, and racist mentality, which fuels and is fueled by the extreme present-day versions of capitalism and materialism it espouses.

Other cultural groups carry their own burdens. The history of an ethnic group's country of origin may be marked by invasions, plagues, famines, natural disasters, or other events that have left burdens on the culture. Immigration, and the reasons for it, also constitute a source of burdens for a group. Many immigrants did not leave their homes by choice; consequently, they are often burdened by intense fears of poverty or political oppression. The wrenching process of cutting family and career ties in the home country and of entering a strange and often hostile culture adds to these burdens. In this regard, the burdens carried by African-Americans are particularly oppressive, since their ancestors were dragged from their tribal homes, brutalized, and enslaved. For this group, then, on top of burdens of fear are layered burdens of rage and power-lessness. To compound this predicament for African-Americans, the culture that imposed these burdens is the dominant culture of the society in which they now live.

Just as with individuals and families, cultural burdens create within ethnic groups imbalances, polarizations and leadership problems. These burdens can also polarize relations between and among groups.

In addition to carrying burdens, each ethnic group carries values and customs that perhaps were adaptive or healthy in the context in which the group evolved, but differ from those of mainstream U.S. culture and vary in terms of how well they fit. That is, just as a sensitive, compassionate child does not fit well into a family where other members are hard-driving and competitive, the cultural characteristics of some ethnic groups do not fit well into a society whose dominant group's values stress competition and mobility. Below, I discuss further mainstream U.S. culture's extremes and the kind of families and individuals it produces, and then discuss some common characteristics of groups that evolved in very different contexts.

The Middle-Class Mainstream U.S. Context

Materialism

First and foremost, the United States is a capitalistic society in which corporations need a large pool of middle-level employees who are willing to put the corporation, and their advancement within it, ahead of the interests of their families of origin or procreation. Needed also are millions of consumers who believe they can derive the intimacy they lack in family life from expensive items they can buy.

To diminish the influence of parts of individuals that value family life, people are bombarded through the mass media with materialistic messages that create a "me-first" culture, where striving for personal success in the form of money or status overrides consideration of relationship networks. As Todd Gitlin (1983) comments,

> Television's world is relentlessly upbeat, clean and materialistic. Even more sweepingly, with few exceptions prime time gives us people preoccupied with personal ambition. If not utterly consumed by ambition and the fear of ending up as losers, these characters take both the ambition and the fear for granted. . . . Personal ambition and consumerism are the driving forces of their lives . . . and this doesn't even take into consideration the incessant commercials, which convey the idea that human aspirations for liberty, pleasure, accomplishment and status can be fulfilled in the realm of consumption. (pp. 268–269)

Geographic and Social Mobility

Another burden of fear was bestowed upon a whole generation of Americans by the Great Depression, which made people willing to sacrifice anything to achieve financial security. For that generation, the most important question when facing a move was "How will this affect my career?", not "How will this affect my marriage or kids or parents?" In their climb up the corporate ladder, families routinely moved, and still move, every 2 or 3 years. As Robert Bellah and his colleagues (Bellah, Madsen, Sullivan, Swidler, & Tipton, 1985) report in *Habits of the Heart*, their hallmark study of mainstream U.S. values, "Being tied to one particular job, in one particular location is tantamount to being stuck, trapped, denied the opportunity for personal fulfillment" (p. 186). The roots of relational networks have barely grown before they are dug up again and transplanted a thousand miles or more away.

Isolation

The isolation resulting from this repeated uprooting tends to reinforce the materialistic parts of family members. As the family is perpetually having to present an image to strangers and gets fewer rewards from emotional connections, issues of status and appearance come to predominate. In turn, the materialistic striving reinforces mobility, which in turn reinforces materialism.

This circular relationship between isolation and materialism was eloquently described in Young and Willmott's (1957) classic study of the effects on families that moved from a highly stable, homogeneous working-class borough in East London to a housing development outside London.

> In Bethnal Green [the borough] people commonly belong to a close network of personal relationships. They know intimately dozens of other local people living near at hand. . . . Common family residence since childhood is the matrix of friendship. In this situation, Bethnal Greeners are not, as we see it, concerned to any marked extent with what is usually thought of as 'status'. It is true of course that people have different kinds of jobs, different kinds of houses. . . . But these attributes are not so important in evaluating others. It is personal characteristics which matter. . . . In a community of long-standing, status, in so far as it is determined by job and income and education, is more or less irrelevant to a person's worth. He is judged instead, if he is judged at all, more in the round, as a person with the usual mixture of all kinds of qualities, some good, some bad, many indefinable. . . . They have the security of belonging to a series of small and overlapping groups, and from their fellows they get the respect they need.
>
> How different is Greenleigh [the development]. Where nearly everyone is a stranger, there is no means of uncovering personality. People cannot be judged by their personal characteristics. . . . Judgement must therefore rest on the trappings of the man rather than on the man himself.

If people have nothing else to go by, they judge from his appearance, his house, or even his Minimotor. . . . The children, in particular, must be well dressed so that neighbors, and even more school-friends and teachers, will think well of them, and of the parents. . . . One might even suggest, to generalize, that the less the personal respect received in small group relationships, the greater is the striving for the kind of impersonal respect embodied in a status judgement. The lonely man, fearing he is looked down on, becomes the acquisitive man; possession the balm of anxiety; anxiety the spur to unfriendliness. (pp. 161–164)

Young and Willmott found this isolation and consequent materialism to be true even of those who had lived in the development for 6 or 7 years, and these people were living next to other Londoners. It is that much more difficult in a heterogeneous society such as the United States to leave a stable network and create a new one, where people often find themselves among very diverse kinds of people. In turn, this isolation increases the dependence on television as the centerpiece of the family, which also in turn increases materialism.

The frequent disconnection from kin or friend networks has other consequences besides materialism. Carol Anderson (1982) reviewed the literature on the effects of family isolation and found them to include decreased marital solidarity; increased rates of mental hospital admissions and consultations with doctors; and increased self-reports of symptoms.

Marital Expectations

In highly mobile middle-class mainstream U.S. culture, children, are expected to leave their parents at an early age, so the only constant relationship amid all these transitional ones is marriage. Thus, in lieu of a stable network of emotionally satisfying relationships, most of people's emotional eggs wind up in the connubial basket. Unlike many other cultures, a spouse is expected to be far more than just a partner in parenthood or in a struggle for economic survival, or a bridge connecting two extended families. The idealized middle-class American marriage is a union of soulmates who have selected each other and who enjoy a consistently high level of intellectual, emotional, and sexual intimacy throughout their long lives together. This glorification of romantic love (and the consequent fear of commitment) can be seen as having resulted, in part, from the burden of great expectations placed on the marital relationship by a highly mobile culture.

This is not to suggest that in more stable, homogeneous contexts, love between spouses is absent as a value. Rather, U.S. mainstream culture has raised the status of love to the point where it is seen as "the major justification for family relations" (Hareven, 1982, p. 456). In addition, the definition of love has been changed to one that fits better within a highly individualistic context. The more traditional view of love, and one that fits better in many ethnic contexts, is that love is something to be worked at and grown over time as each person becomes increasingly willing to sacrifice for the partner. As Bellah et al. (1985) put it, "Love thus becomes a matter of will and action rather than of feelings. While one cannot coerce one's feelings, one can learn to obey God's commands and to love others in a selfless way" (p. 94).

In contrast, a kind of selfishness is essential to U.S. middle-class love. People believe that in order to love another, they must love and assert themselves. The kind of self-sacrificial or obligatory thinking that is the cornerstone of traditional love is seen as leading to excessive dependence (codependence) or suffocation by mainstream Americans, who do not want to be constrained by family obligations from partaking fully of the good life. Ideally, one stays with a partner because that person satisfies one more than any other does; if that were to change, one should be able to change partners.

In sum, middle-class marriage in the United States carries not only unprecedented emotional expectations, but also an unprecedented lack of traditional obligation. All this is in keeping with the previously mentioned need in a capitalistic society for a willingness to put materialistic and achievement-oriented values before family commitments or considerations. Bellah et al. (1985) interviewed a man named Brian, who exemplifies this ethic:

> Still rising toward the peak of a career that has defined his identity by its progress, Brian looks back on his twenties and thirties, devoted to advancing his career at the expense of tending his marriage and family life, and concedes, "I got totally swept up in my own progress, in promotions and financial successes." Yet even now, Brian's definition of success revolves around an open-ended career on the upswing. . . . "Where I come as close as I can to performing at the absolute limits of my capacity. That's success." (p. 68)

In the face of a multitude of Brians and a culture that reinforces them, love and marriage must accommodate themselves accordingly.

Ambitious, Autonomous Children

In a stable ethnic network, in which there is little opportunity for or tradition of economic or geographic movement, children do not leave home in the mainstream American sense, and their parents' nest is never empty. To socialize children in such contexts for personal ambition and independence is either to prepare them for a life of frustration, or to threaten the future of the network if they were to act on those values and leave. Thus, many ethnic parents raise their children to be obedient, loyal, and conforming, and to put the good of the family well before any personal desires. These families are generally characterized by an authority-based parenting style. Children often wind up doing and thinking the same things as their parents.

In contrast, an American middle-class child is not to become a parental replica. Rather, he or she should be a "seeker after success and love, ready to venture far from parental patterns in search of those ends" (Bellah et al., 1985, p. 60). More than in any other culture, child rearing in mainstream U.S. culture encourages children to negotiate with parents for what they want, to compete with peers in all arenas, to desire and expect material possessions, to solve problems on their own, and not to rely on tradition or authority. These children are also expected to leave home as young adults, and to enter and succeed in a harsh, survival-of-the-fittest economy. In many ways, their childhood is a long proving and training ground for this reality.

Extrafamilial Relations

The intense loyalty to one's extended family that is commonly nurtured in stable, homogeneous networks often includes a fear or distrust of the extrafamilial, and strong proscriptions against getting too close to anyone who is not "family" or at least not of the same ethnicity. These thick boundaries around one's immediate family or ethnic group have survival value in cases where the crossing of the boundaries could mean the dissolution of intricate webs of social obligation and tradition. In the United States, many formerly distinct cultures have diffused into oblivion as they have been caught up in the powerful currents of the mainstream.

Present-day middle-class Americans, on the other hand, already have little concern for social obligation or tradition, and so are less constrained from mingling with unrelated people. Indeed, since they move so frequently to strange neighborhoods, they need to be able to create new support networks quickly but not to become too attached emotionally to the people in them, since no one knows when anyone will be moving on. Thus, mainstream Americans learn a friendly style of relating that allows some degree of quick acquaintance-level connection to compatible networks through work or through community or school organizations.

Also, U.S. capitalism fosters such a style of relating, because in many cases friends are also potential clients or contacts. Because everyone might secretly be making a sale, however, it is hard to trust the sincerity of anyone's friendliness. Since people are all selling themselves, it also becomes terribly important to look attractive or stylish. This pressure regarding appearances gives the perfectionistically evaluative parts of individuals prominence, so that they are constantly judging themselves and others by how they look. In this climate, it is difficult to create an emotionally satisfying network of friends.

Isolation is another by-product of our competitiveness. Since the Industrial Revolution of the first half of the 19th century, which separated the home from the workplace, Americans have viewed their homes as havens in a heartless world (Hareven, 1982). Whereas in many ethnic contexts homes and neighborhoods are the center of a great deal of social activity, American middle-class homes are seen as private retreats—the only places where their owners can find respite from the selfish, competitive, and immoral jungle.

Since that time and until recently, the primary role of a wife was to be the custodian of this therapeutic refuge. As such, she was expected, through her domestic talents, to create a stress-free, loving, nurturant household environment in which her husband, the weary warrior, could lick his wounds and gird for the next day's battle. Although the prohibition from entering the working world that kept women isolated in these little castles has lifted, the other expectations derived from this "cult of domesticity" remain. Thus it is very possible (and, unless a family possesses the requisite social skills and initiative, it is likely) for many families to live highly isolated lives, even though they dwell in densely populated middle-class communities. It is also likely for the wives in these families to be overburdened as well as isolated.

Anxiety

Most mainstream Americans could use some kind of haven because their world does indeed seem heartless, and they often stand alone against it. Even in the 19th century, social commentators such as the French author Alexis de Tocqueville could see that Americans were unusually anxious and insecure. de Tocqueville attributed this condition, in part, to the constant striving to take full advantage of this land of opportunity:

> I have seen the freest and best educated of men in circumstances the happiest to be found in the world; yet it seemed to me that a cloud habitually hung on their brow, and they seemed serious and almost sad even in their pleasures [because they] never stop thinking about the good things they have not got. (quoted in Bellah et al., 1985, p. 117)

This is a vivid description of the striving, acquisitive parts that dominate so many middle-class Americans today.

In addition, in the capitalistic free market people were freer than ever to fail, particularly before the federal safety nets were installed after the Great Depression. Without solid kinship or friendship networks, failure spelled disaster. Thus, the mainstream U.S. striving for success is driven as much by fear as it is by the profit motive. One never knows when the market will shift or a competitor will get an edge and suddenly all will be lost. As Bellah et al. (1985) state,

> Just when he could count on fewer and fewer people for "unconditional acceptance," the individual had to be self-disciplined, competitive, ambitious, able to respond to rapidly changing situations and demands, able to leave home to go to school and follow the opportunities of professional advancement. It was under these conditions that a concern for mental health became a central American preoccupation and a wide variety of therapeutic nostrums appeared. (p. 120)

Seen in this cultural context, the models of therapy that have evolved in an attempt to help these anxious Americans reinforce many of the same values that create their anxiety. Many therapies have accepted the goal of trying to help people and families adapt to mainstream American culture, without questioning whether the culture itself is healthy. Nearly all forms of therapy in the United States are designed to reduce what is considered to be the anachronistic sense of social obligation or guilt that constrains clients from achieving their full potential or expressing themselves. We have been helping people shed baggage and streamline, so that they can compete more successfully.

Summary

The pioneers' hard-edged individualism created the context for U.S. corporate capitalistic economy and culture. The values that have co-evolved within this context—materialism; personal ambition over family considerations; romantic love as the basis for marriage; democratic parenting style; mobility and independence; home as a haven; and a friendly but not emotionally involved style of sociability—are the values that fit best with and perpetuate the context, and are very different from values in other cultural contexts.

Accordingly, the family structure that fits best with middle-class mainstream U.S. values and context is the streamlined nuclear model, in which the parents' primary alliance is with each other; grandparents only advise or provide support, and do so from a distance; and children are raised to be competitive, ambitious, and self-reliant. Families that evolve such a structure have the best chance of "functioning" in this context, and the goal of family therapy, after all, has been to make families "functional." Families that have not made the enormous structural transformation required by this context are likely to show all manner of "pathology" in their communication and behavior.

The point I am trying to make is that mainstream U.S. culture is highly imbalanced because of historical burdens that elevated the striving, individualistic parts of its leaders. "Hyper-Americanized" families and individuals become microcosms of these imbalances, and in turn perpetuate them in the culture. That is, such families are emotionally isolated; are dominated by the managerial coalition of striving, evaluative, and entitled parts; show little tolerance for weakness or imperfection; and have little time or inclination for intimacy. The internal systems of hyper-Americanized individuals reflect these imbalances and polarizations. A problem or syndrome (e.g., bulimia) in a hyper-Americanized family is treated very differently and has different qualities than in an ethnic family dominated by more traditional values.

Traditional Ethnic Contexts

Cultures around the world vary considerably in their values and family structures, and much has been written regarding these differences (Falicov, 1983; McGoldrick, Pearce, & Giordano, 1982). I believe, however, that the values and family structures that have evolved in communities that have remained relatively stable and ethnically homogeneous over generations or centuries share many fundamental elements, and are very different from the hyper-Americanized values and structure described in the preceding section. Animal species evolving in certain climates, terrains, and predatorial conditions will have some basic characteristics in common with those of other species evolving in similar environments in other parts of the planet, and different from those of species evolving in very different conditions. The evolution of values and family structure is no different. In this section, I highlight the values and aspects of family structure that conflict most with the middle-class mainstream U.S. context. Most of these generalizations apply primarily to the rural or nonmodernized ethnic contexts in which most of the world's cultures have evolved.

Low Mobility

In a setting where people do not move up economically or away geographically, individualistic ambition creates either frustration with or desertion from the community. The survival and perpetuation of the network depend on the cohesiveness of its members. If young people leave, no one remains to support the elderly or to replace the services and trades that go with them. Thus, the importance of loyalty to the clan and to its traditions are stressed over interests in personal advancement.

Family Reputation

In addition to not straying far from the nest, younger members of such networks are under constant pressure to maintain their families' good reputation or image, which generally means not deviating from traditional male or female roles within the ethnic network. This pressure comes in part from living in close proximity, so that it feels as if a hundred eyes are on each person as he or she walks down the street. In addition, however, in many cultures the one way for a family to advance is for a child to marry someone from a wealthier family. The primary determinant of such a marriage is the family's reputation. In the relatively impersonal, anonymous middle-class U.S. context, family reputation is not nearly as important for advancement, so children are permitted more room for individuality.

Marital Expectations

In many ethnic contexts, it is often more difficult and less necessary to have a marriage in which a spouse is the primary source of emotional fulfillment, as in the ideal middle-class U.S. marriage described above. It is more difficult because, amid such proximity to relatives, it is harder for a couple to avoid involving relatives in disputes; it is also harder to shift primary alliances from parent to spouse if one never moves, and consequently never creates a break in dependence or closeness. As Falicov and Brudner-White (1983) state, "the extended family tends to discourage the elevation of the marital tie above all others because this threatens the ideal of continuity between the generations, a value so central to extended family life" (p. 55).

Marital primacy is also less necessary because there are many other alternatives to marital closeness for each spouse. As Young and Willmott (1957) wrote of the families that remained in East London, "They have remained in their district and consequently in their families of origin. The wife stays close to her mother because she already shares so many common interests and associations, an since she stays nearby, she keeps them alive and renews them" (p. 117). Similarly, in many cultures, husbands remain part of an "*amigo* system," or spend time with male work friends or with their fathers, or brothers. The couple's children provide another convenient and never-ending focus for emotional investment. In addition, the roles of each spouse are clearly defined and distinct from each other in many ethnic networks, so that there is less need for cooperation, collaboration, or mutual decision making. There is plenty of help and advice available from the extended family, so that spouses have to rely less on each other.

Thus marriage is neither expected nor able to be what hyper-Americanized marriage is supposed to be. This is not to suggest that such relationships are barren of love, but that the love within them is of a different nature. It stems less from self-awareness and disclosure, and more from the connectedness that comes with working hard for common family goals or from the sense of well-being that comes with fitting snugly into a larger system. For these reasons, then, in such contexts it is common that each spouse's primary emotional attachment will be cross-generational (i.e., to a parent or a child) rather than marital.

Summary

To summarize this section, the family values and structure that tend to evolve in ethnic contexts are, for good reason, quite different from those of the middle-class mainstream U.S. context. Extended family networks are likely to value loyalty, selflessness, and tradition over personal ambition or autonomy; family reputation and role adherence over individuality; an emphasis on relationships and network connectedness over materialism; and a sense of staying with one's own kind over American-style sociability. Family structure is more likely to stress cross-generational primacy over marital primacy; authority over democratic parenting style; a wide range of family leaders rather than just the parents; and relatively rigid boundaries between the families and the nonfamilial.

Many families in the United States remain within the ethnic networks and communities that characterize many American cities. There they can protect traditional values and customs from the onrushing waves of hyper-Americanicanized values. But while remaining in their ethnic communities, they also suffer from the racism and prejudice with which the dominant majority has burdened them. Their opportunities are constrained, and polarizations often develop between generations as the younger members chafe at these constraints, become more worried about their future, and thus become more eager to fit in.

Transitional Families

Thus, families leave these ethnic "islands" and try to swim along with the other families in the U.S. mainstream. Unfortunately, many of these families are not equipped to survive amid the competitive, isolating currents, and are not immune to the toxic values that pollute the waters. Studies of specific ethnic groups that compared those living within the ethnic groups' communities to those living outside those ethnic enclaves found higher hospital admissions for schizophrenia in the outside-dwelling groups (Mintz & Schwartz, 1964; Rabkin, 1979; Wechsler & Pugh, 1967). To function in the mainstream without becoming severely symptomatic, these families need to transform themselves into the streamlined, mobile American units described earlier. This is often not possible, although it is what many family therapists attempt. Even when such a transformation is relatively successful, a family is likely to accumulate burdens of resentment and shame, as its ripping away from the extended network leaves open sores that may never heal.

Thus, ethnic families that have left their enclaves (what I call "transitional families") are at great risk of becoming isolated and child-focused. This is because the parents have few emotional outlets other than the children. They no longer have their same-sex networks, and they are not oriented toward getting intimacy from their marriages (which, because of the isolation, are carrying an untenable burden anyway). On top of this, they are likely either to carry the burden of patriarchal attitudes as a residue from the ethnic enclave or to adopt the current U.S. version of such attitudes, in which women are supposed to both keep the haven *and* bring home money. For these reasons, transitional families are at great risk. They often appear to be extremely enmeshed—emotionally reactive and controlling—especially as the time approaches when children should, according to mainstream U.S. standards, become more emotionally and geographically distant.

In a case where a husband and wife come from different (or even polarized) ethnic groups, all of these issues are compounded by two additional burdens on the marriage. The first is the clash of cultures within the marriage. The second is disapproval from each spouse's family of origin and, in some cases, from the mainstream culture. These extra burdens add to such a family's sense of alienation and internal tension.

Transitional families are not just those in which parents are the ones who left the old country or the ethnic community. Many families remain in this transitional state for generations and suffer as a result. These families are frozen in time, in much the same way that parts of traumatized people are stuck in the past. The hallmark of a transitional family, then, is the lack of fit between its values or structure and the culture in which it exists.

Taxonomy of Families

Now we can construct a taxonomy of families in the United States:

1. Tradition-based families, which live in ethnic communities and struggle to preserve their traditional values.

2. Transitional families which live in the U.S. mainstream and have adopted some of the mainstream's values, but have not fully shed their ethnic values and structure.
3. Hyper-Americanized families, which live in and fit with the mainstream, and have absorbed high levels of middle-class U.S. values.

This taxonomy is admittedly oversimplified and incomplete, but it can help a therapist and family members understand the cultural context of a given family's circumstances. A family will have different kinds of imbalances, polarizations, and leadership problems, depending on which of these three categories it fits into.

To help the reader organize all these ideas about culture, let us return to the perspective of constraints. As the reader will recall, a client is kept from achieving balanced, harmonious Self-leadership by burdens accrued over time and by living in a constraining environment. This chapter thus far has expanded our perspective on these burdens and this constraining environment beyond the idiosyncratic traumas the client has experienced or the peculiarities of his or her family. The client's constraints will also be related to the ethnic group he or she is born into; the burdens that ethnic group carries; its relationship to the dominant culture; and whether the client's family is tradition-based, transitional, or hyper-Americanized.

Contrasting Transitional and Hyper-Americanized Families

To illustrate how different cultural predicaments constrain people differently, I now compare two bulimic clients in their late teens. Sophia was raised in a transitional family. Her parents grew up in the Greek Town neighborhood of Chicago; her father earned a law degree and found a good job, and after her parents married they moved into a mainstream northern suburb. Sara's family, on the other hand, had been in the mainstream for generations. Her father worked for a large corporation and the family moved around the Midwest for years, finally settling in a Chicago suburb. I begin with Sophia's story and then contrast it to Sara's.

Sophia's Family

Background

Sophia D was a 17-year-old high school senior who had been severely bulimic for 6 months. Her parents had little contact with her extended family, which remained in Greek Town. When Mr. and Mrs. D first left the neighborhood, everyone in their respective families seemed proud of both of them and supportive of their moving onward and upward, except for Mrs. D's mother, who wanted them to live nearby.

The suburb they moved to was almost an hour's drive from Greek Town, and Mr. D wanted his wife to stay home with Sophia. She complied despite her sense of loneliness and alienation from her neighbors, who mostly seemed to stay in their homes—or, if they did venture out, dressed up even to go grocery shopping. Mrs. D tried to maintain close contact with her mother and sisters and phoned them frequently, but the trek into Greek Town with Sophia was too much to make more than once a week, and there was so much housework if they were to keep up appearances in the new neighborhood. She also sensed that the family and friends they had left now saw her as different, as if her money and new status were getting in the way.

As an aspiring young lawyer, Mr. D had to work long hours to compete with his colleagues and had little time for his new family, much less for maintaining ties to his old friends and family. He found his wife's sadness and her demands for more of his time confusing and oppressive, since he spent every spare minute with her and Sophia. Besides, she seemed to enjoy the money he was making. She spent it like crazy, redecorating repeatedly because she wanted her home to look perfect. Mr. D took Mrs. D to a psychiatrist, who diagnosed postpartum depression and medicated her.

Both parents lived for Sophia, whom they expected to excel in school, and also to be highly obedient and loyal. Depressed and isolated, Mrs. D kept her daughter with her always when she was not in school, and took special pride in Sophia's cheerful and polite demeanor. This began to change as Sophia entered adolescence. The parents, who tried to maintain some of their Greek traditions and identity, were chagrinned by Sophia's decreasing interest in her heritage. Mrs. D was embarrassed by Sophia's style of dress and manners, particularly when they were around members of her family (who, as Mrs. D knew, had concerns about her parenting). Mrs. D and Sophia began to fight over what the mother considered her daughter's excessive vanity and eating habits. Mrs. D viewed feeding her family as one of her most important jobs. She cooked the way her own mother did, and she expected her family to appreciate and eat the food.

Sophia was "Daddy's little girl" until she stopped being so little or girlish, at which point he abruptly stopped spending much time with her and seemed uneasy in her presence. Mr. D maintained a patriarchal style around the house with both his wife and his daughter. But when the two women fought he was likely to side with Sophia, since both he and his daughter were bothered by Mrs. D's nagging attempts to change them. They shared a belief that Mrs. D was too old-fashioned and was trying to hold on to the past.

Both parents were also extremely protective of Sophia, compared to her friends' parents. Mrs. D would search Sophia's room for evidence of misbehavior as Sophia began to go out with friends. Her father alternated between defending her right to privacy and joining his wife in scare tactics about the outside world.

When the family entered therapy, the fights between Sophia and her mother had escalated to the point of being almost constant and sometimes physical. Because of the bulimia, the fights currently focused on Sophia's eating behavior, with Mrs. D hounding her daughter to stop wasting all their food and to show more self-control. Mrs. D seemed almost comically obsessed by Sophia's eating, while Mr. D (who by this time had high blood pressure and angina) again alternated between trying to get his wife to let up and disdaining his daughter's disgusting behavior.

Sophia had become withdrawn, sullen, and sneaky at home; on the rare occasions when she went out, she was drinking heavily with friends. The parents agreed that Sophia was in no shape to go away to college the next year. Although she protested that they were wrong, Sophia herself seemed to have mixed feelings about leaving home.

The Transitional Family's Predicament

A Family without a Culture. Sophia's family illustrates many themes common to transitional families with whom I have worked. Mr. and Mrs. D carried the burden of emotional cutoff from their extended family. Yet one or both still saw aspects of mainstream U.S. culture as threatening and were disturbed by its influence on their child. Many of their protective and intrusive behaviors were related to fears of losing their daughter to this strange culture; yet they no longer had the support of a network of relatives to enforce their sanctions, and felt that Sophia needed to be somewhat American to succeed.

Father–Daughter Coalitions. In addition, coalitions between the father and daughter against the mother were common for many reasons, all related to the burden of patriarchy. First, Mrs. D was largely responsible for her daughter's socialization, and so was more involved in trying to shape her behavior through daily critiques of her dressing, eating, or cleaning habits. Second, Mr. D's approval was highly regarded and competed for by both women in the family. The father was still highly solicitous of his "little girl" at times, so she was reluctant to cross him and lose her special position. Third, Mr. D occasionally defended Sophia from Mrs. D's intrusiveness, and blamed his wife for their daughter's problems. Finally, because the mother's position was so bleak, she came to use her daughter as her source of intimacy or distraction from her exiles. Although parts of Sophia accepted this burden, other parts resented it and reacted to the mother from this resentment.

Marital Tension. Similarly, as noted earlier, the parents' marriage in many transitional families is not structured for the isolation of nucleari-zation; as a result, there is often a secret and growing tension between parents. This tension can create the need for a distraction. In the D family's case, Sophia was the one available to carry the burden of protecting the parental marriage. Consider the following dialogue be-tween Mrs. D and the therapist:

THERAPIST: Sophia says that she's very worried about you and about your husband. She thinks that your marriage wouldn't make it if she grew up.

MOTHER: That's crazy. Why should she worry about our marriage? Nobody's happy all the time.

THERAPIST: She says she doesn't worry about you two splitting up. She doesn't think there's much chance of that. She thinks you will be sad. You have been a mother a long time. She worries that soon she will be gone, and then what will you do?

MOTHER: That's crazy. I don't want her worrying about me—she has her own problems. I never worried about my mother. She had 10 kids and they never worried about her.

THERAPIST: Was your mother's mother around then? And her sisters and friends?

MOTHER: Yes.

THERAPIST: Then no wonder you didn't have to worry about her. Is your mother available to you, or your siblings or cousins?

MOTHER: No, not much any more.

THERAPIST: Do you have many friends?

MOTHER: I see what you're getting at, but I don't want Sophia to worry about me. She has her own life to think of.

The Mother's Predicament. The exchange above illustrates not only the predicament in which many women in traditional families find themselves, but also the difficulty they have discussing their feelings about this predicament. They are constrained by the family burden encouraging selflessness and sacrifice and discouraging assertiveness, particularly in women, and by their parts that constantly remind them of the rule.

Thus, in many ways Mrs. D was in the loneliest, most unenviable position in her family. She was isolated from her female network; estranged from her husband; given primary responsibility for the impossible job of keeping Sophia thinking and acting according to ethnic values; and blamed by Sophia, her husband, and her own parents for daughter's problems. She felt dependent on Sophia for some sort of closeness, yet resented and envied her daughter's special relationship with her husband.

For many women in this isolated position, domestic duties, which would have been one of their prominent roles in the ethnic network, become their obsession. Having few other sources of esteem, a mother invests heavily in how well she cooks and how well her family eats. Thus, in the absence of more direct forms of communication, food and what family members do with it become one of the most important arenas for defining relationships. In Sophia's, she could demonstrate her love for, or at least acquiescence to, her mother by eating heartily. Similarly, she could express her disdain for or rebellion against her mother by not eating, or, worse, eating and then vomiting what had been eaten.

In addition to being perceived as a rejection of the mother, this squandering of what has already been eaten is particularly contemptible and inconceivable to transitional families, many of which come from backgrounds of scarcity and carry those burdens. Some parents' extraordinary revulsion toward bulimia makes more sense in that light. A bulimic daughter is torn between conflicting pressures. To please her parents, she must eat a lot; however, to feel acceptable with her peers and her culture, she must diet so as to be thin. Thus, her eating and weight take on an additional layer of meaning, defining whether her loyalties lie with her family or with mainstream U.S. culture.

The Father's Predicament. Many fathers in such families have little experience relating to women as equals. A father may derive traditional, patriarchal attitudes from his ethnic culture that are accentuated by his frustration over being unable to satisfy his isolated wife. Not knowing how else to relate when she is upset with him, he tends to intensify patronizing, instrumental problem-solving attempts or authoritarian commands for her to "straighten up."

As in many cases, the most intimacy in Mr. D's life came when Sophia was a little girl and he could hold, comfort, and nurture her without feeling afraid of his sexuality. They had a special relationship that he missed and, particularly at times of stress, wanted to recreate. Sophia's problems frustrated him. When she could not follow his orders to use will power to stop the binge–purge episodes, he felt personally rejected, as if he had lost his authority or his position as her hero. Along these lines, a father like Mr. D may have trouble accepting a therapist who may succeed where he is failing. The result of these conflicting feelings or parts of such a father is that he is likely to vacillate among protective parts, one minute withdrawing from and giving up on his daughter, the next minute angrily commanding that she change, and then the next trying to evoke their past "Daddy's girl" closeness.

Selfishness and Distrust of the Extrafamilial. Underscoring all of the rules and beliefs described thus far is the sense that directly asking for something for oneself, or refusing a family request, is the cardinal family sin of being selfish. This family-comes-first antiassertiveness can be used by families who are isolated from a network to keep family members stuck together. Thus, a daughter's desire to leave home (or in some families even to date) becomes selfish; her refusal to do more things with her mother is selfish; her bingeing is selfish, as is her refusal of food when she is dieting; and so on. This rule against self-assertion also blocks direct communicating about differences, preventing their resolution.

Whereas the isolation of hyper-Americanized families is maintained by competitiveness, transitional families often carry a strong distrust of the extrafamilial. This fear of the outside world not only perpetuates their isolation, but also presents a boundary that is difficult for the American-ized therapist to penetrate. It also makes protective parts of the bulimic daughter fearful to the point where she often has trouble trusting and getting close to peers, which increases her reliance on bingeing.

Sara's Family

Background

Sara B had been bulimic for 2 years before her parents found out. For Mr. B this was a bolt out of the blue, because he had thought everything was perfect for Sara. And, as he frequently told her, he couldn't understand why she couldn't exercise some self-control and just quit. Mrs. B had seen some signs that Sara was having eating problems, but didn't say anything for fear of embarrassing Sara and upsetting her husband. She now alternated between bouts of guilt and rage, fighting frequently with Sara over food.

Sara hated the way she looked, particularly her weight, and felt ashamed for bringing such a disgusting problem into her parents' life. At the same time, she blamed her mother's concern with appearances for contributing to her problem. Preoccupied with worries about aging, Mrs. B had had plastic surgery on her body and face. Sara complained that whenever she went out with her mother, Mrs. B urged her to dress well, but always made sure that she (Mrs. B) looked a little better. Sara also complained that her mother intruded into her life and tried to control her, especially now that the eating problem was overt.

Having taken the role of helping her husband be a successful sales manager by managing the perfect household, Mrs. B now felt like a failure. For the past 17 years, taking care of Sara had been Mrs. B's primary job, and now her worst suspicions about her mothering were confirmed by Sara's embarrassing problem. Her tremendous desire for her daughter to get well was an expression of concern not only for Sara's health, but also for the health of her own self-concept. Out of shame, Mrs. B had told no one, not even her own family, about Sara's problem. She never confided in any of her friends about personal issues, knowing that when they gossiped about someone outside their circle who had problems with a child, they often implied that "it figured, knowing the parents."

Mr. B's job was extremely stressful and competitive, with little reward other than money, so he looked to his family as his source of pride and enjoyment. Because of this, Sara's problems and the conflicts they generated were very distressing for him. If his family was a failure, then what did he have to live for? The more distressed Mr. B became, the more both Mrs. B and Sara believed they were failing him, and fought with each other.

The striving and perfectionistic parts that dominated Mr. and Mrs. B and Sara had kept them from getting close to one another, and kept them on the run from their own (and each other's) sad and lonely parts. Their lives of quiet and denied desperation required culturally sanctioned analgesics: food for Sara; work and alcohol for Mr. B; possessions and pursuit of beauty for Mrs. B. All of them became increasingly desperate for feedback to counter their sense of emptiness and unworthiness. Mrs. B needed to know that she was still attractive to men, and that she had a better house, husband, and haircut than her friends. Mr. B needed to be the best salesman in the computer software corporation he worked for. Sara craved the approval of her father, who rarely gave it to her despite her high level of academic achievement.

The weight of her parents' (especially her father's) disappointment and shame had made Sara hide her bulimia for 2 years. Once the bulimia was discovered, Sara often felt that her mother's only concern was how her problem looked to others, and that her father's main worry was that the family therapy appointments interfered with his work schedule. Like her mother, Sara was too ashamed to tell any of her friends about her problem. She had withdrawn from the battle for status that took place daily at her high school, and now spent most of her time in her room.

In comparing Sara's family to Sophia's, it is interesting to see how, despite the different burdens carried by the two families, they wound up in similar predicaments and patterns. Both families were isolated, highly concerned about appearances, and rigidly polarized. The reasons for these characteristics and the issues around which they revolved were quite different, but many patterns were the same.

The Hyper-Americanized Family's Predicament

Patriarchy, Appearances, and Materialism. Sara's family had been steeped for years in the mainstream U.S. values of materialism, competitiveness, and obsession with a youthful, beautiful appearance. Like Sophia's family, Sara's also was patriarchal, as reflected mainly in two arenas. The first was in their deference to the demands of Mr. B's career. Since it was a primary source of money, the family acquiesced to whatever sacrifice the father's job demanded—and it demanded a great deal. Like most hyper-Americanized men, Mr. B worked long hours; even when he was home, his achievement parts were still running, keeping him distracted and unavailable. He also expected and received more access to opportunities for recreation or relaxation than Mrs. B did.

Mrs. B was like many hyper-Americanized mothers in being lonely and frustrated with this situation (although many only acknowledge these feelings late in therapy). She suffered in silence, in some cases between infrequent outbursts of rage, because she, like her husband, subscribed to the family's governing materialistic ethic. Parts of her were willing to put up with a barren marriage and imbalances in domestic responsibility and influence, so as to maintain the family's life style and social status. She also found that her husband tended to recoil from her expressions of unhappiness.

The second patriarchal arena was related to the pressure on the women in the family to appear attractive to men. Both parents made frequent comments regarding their daughter's weight, but, because the father represented the successful male's perspective and because he had high status in the family, his comments hit hard. Mrs. B, of course, was hyperconcerned about and critical of her own weight, in addition to her daughter's, and focused her achievement parts on dieting. She knew her husband liked thin women, and as she aged, it became increasingly important to her to keep a man-pleasing figure.

Being Thin to Win. Thus, from a young age, Sara was taught that being fashionably thin was desperately important, that attracting a successful man was her ticket to a happy life, and that people would value her primarily for how she looked. In many hyper-Americanized families, females are conscious of and competitive about how much they eat at mealtimes, and discussion of food and diets consumes an inordinate percentage of family conversation. This weight rivalry often veils a general competition for a father's approval. It is not uncommon for a bulimic daughter to express the belief that she is her father's favorite, partly because of her appearance, and that she feels her mother resents and tries to undermine her relationship with her father for this reason.

Keeping Up Appearances Equals Denial. Although these patriarchal and materialistic imbalances created tense coalitions in the B family, these tensions lurked beneath a surface of apparent propriety and closeness that the family tried to maintain at any cost. In keeping with U.S. corporate culture's fear of losing one's competitive edge by appearing weak, unattractive, or imperfect, members of hyper-Americanized families try to hide their conflicts from the outside world, from one another, and from themselves. They are dominated by the "power of positive thinking"; complaints about the family's structure, or expressions of sadness or loneliness, are disdained as negative thinking and become the "exiles" in the family. People should be able to do or feel anything if they have enough will power, so if a family member has a problem, it means that the person has a lack of will. Fat people are viewed as extremely weak-willed and repulsive. (The exception to this rule is physical disease, which is seen as out of a person's control. For this reason, it is not surprising that many bulimic clients and other family members become quite attached to the disease metaphor for bulimia.)

This cloud of denial is perhaps the most pernicious by-product of hyper-Americanized values. In this survival-of-the-fittest culture, the fittest are the flawless. Middle-class Americans are taught to present to the world a seamless exterior; to hide their "weaknesses" and to "never let 'em see you sweat"; to pretend that they have no problems, pain, or blemishes. As Dan had told Sara at one point, "Selling yourself is what life is all about." And people do not buy flawed merchandise. This pretend-we're-perfect philosophy comes to dominate not only the way family members present themselves to the outside world, but also the way they relate to one another.

In such an environment, family members not only deny their feelings—pushing away the parts of them that feel sad, scared, bored, lonely, or angry—but also criticize themselves (and each other) for having such feelings. In these families, bulimic daughters are terribly ashamed of what they do, often go to great lengths to hide their bulimia, and are desperately afraid that they will be discovered. Despite efforts to cover up, many of the hyper-Americanized families I have treated knew of the problem, but didn't speak about it before it came undeniably to the surface.

Often, however, parts of these young women want to break through their families's denial; they are tired of pretending and want their distress to be acknowledged. Some of these clients, therefore, make their symptoms highly visible once their secret has been exposed, as if vowing that their distress will never be denied again. Or clients vacillate between secret and flagrant bingeing, depending on which of their parts have taken over and how their families are reacting.

Frequently, a bulimic daughter is not the only family member who, at least occasionally, tarnishes the perfect family image. Pressure to be perfect cannot always prevent covert conflicts from surfacing or sadness from showing. When family members succumb to such impulses, they often do so in extreme ways because the parts that break through are extreme from having been suppressed, and because everyone else is so afraid of such episodes and reacts so strongly to them. These outbreaks of emotion are commonly followed by attempts to minimize or deny them, or by angry sanctions toward a family member who can be construed as having triggered them. For example, if Mrs. B, in the middle of a spat with Sara, broke into tears and talked of how unhappy her life was, Mr. B would become furious at Sara for having upset her mother.

It is difficult to survive in such families without some kind of distraction or method of self-numbing—some kind of firefighter activity. It is not uncommon to find heavy use of alcohol or tranquilizers in parents and drug abuse in siblings. In addition, once the clients' bulimia is exposed, it frequently becomes a focus of concern or disdain that serves to distract from the families's pervasive tension and fear, as described in Chapters 6 and 7.

The Mother's Predicament. Just as in transitional families, mothers in hyper-Americanized families are lonely and unhappy, but are afraid to express this directly. As a result, they also become highly involved in their daughters' lives. Many of my hyper-Americanized bulimic clients report that from a young age they have acted as their mothers' confidantes, therapists, or companions, and feel responsible for the mother's happiness. They try to comfort and cheer up their mothers more often than vice versa. In addition, these clients feel like failures because they cannot remove their mothers' abiding unhappiness. Commonly, a bulimic daughter reports having warring parts that feel a confusing mixture of guilt over her inability to improve her mother's chronic malaise, resentment that her mother is so preoccupied and emotionally unavailable, and more guilt at the thought that she has stolen her father from her mother.

Mothers also report a range of conflicts. They are concerned about their daughters' health, and frustrated by the daughters' irresponsibility and inability to control themselves. They assume (and are often given by their husbands) primary culpability for their daughters' bulimia, so they are highly bothered by it and determined to change it.

This mixture of extreme parts in the mother–daughter relationship is usually quite combustible. For example, fights erupted quickly between Mrs. B and Sara over picky issues such as eating, dressing, or cleaning. These fights were more bitter when Sara was also involved in protecting her father from her mother or was in competition with her mother for her father's approval. In such cases, the picky issues are surrogates for other intense and threatening issues.

The Daughter's Predicament. Daughters in these hyper-Americanized families come to see their female peers as competitors and male peers as potential mates; consequently, like Sara, they have few real friends with whom they can discuss their distress. A part of them believes that they must find a man to take care of them. That part makes them feel great when they get romantic attention from a man, or when they lose weight as a step toward getting such attention. Conversely, this part makes them feel terrible when they do not get such attention or when they gain weight.

In addition, these daughters are given conflicting mandates regarding what their life goals should be. Consistent with the perfect family image, they are pushed to achieve in school, and yet are taught to be "nice" (nonthreatening, nonassertive, nonintellectual) to avoid scaring away the right kind of man. This socialization process elevates their achievement-oriented parts, but narrows the range of focus for these competitive urges to appearance or school. Other parts that encourage a passive, approval-seeking approach to life are also elevated through this kind of parenting.

Father–daughter relationships often revolve around achievement. For example, Sara reported her accomplishments to her father as a major mode of relating to him. Because Mr. B was often absent or distracted, his attention was a rare commodity, and one way to gain it was to accomplish. Parts of Sara desperately wanted a different, more accepting and nurturing relationship with her father, and believed that if Sara performed well enough she might get some of that. This made for perfectionistic internal standards for achievement, and thus for brutal self-criticism when the standards were not realized. Sara found that after the bulimia was revealed, it became another avenue to her father's attention. In addition, if she couldn't keep up to speed with achieving, having an illness was a convenient excuse.

Bulimia as a Multipurpose Syndrome. To summarize, both Sara and her parents were constrained by their cultural predicament, which influenced their external and internal families toward imbalance and polarization. More specifically, because Sara had little nurturance from either parent and instead often carried the burden of taking care of them, she had a number of parts she had to exile that felt hurt, scared, and empty. Sara's managers learned from her environment to keep her away from her exiles through denying their existence, through studying and shopping constantly, and through being obsessed with her weight. Her firefighters looked to food binges partly because her managers had her starving herself, and consequently created polarizations in the opposite direction. In addition, Sara recalled that whenever she had been upset as a child, her mother had given her some ice cream or candy, so she had learned to look for comestible instead of personal comfort.

This internal family structure was reinforced by the distractive role that her bulimia took on within her external family. It provided an arena for family fights; it reassured Sara and her family that she was a long way from growing up and living independently; and it was a convenient rationale to explain her shifting moods (as her exiles tried to break through the denial) and her less-than-perfect performance. The bingeing was also a way in which some parts could rebel against her diet-crazed parents and their internal representatives, which dominated her psyche. Finally, it was a way for Sara to get some nurturant attention from her parents.

As the preceding two paragraphs indicate, it is simplistic to speak of one purpose or cause of most chronic problems, because they are multipurpose and multicausal. Commonplace notions, such as the idea that Sara binged because she wanted attention or because she was rebelling against her parents, are partially true. It is also true that Sara binged because she wanted to avoid painful feelings or because she starved herself at other times. A syndrome like bulimia has many causes and purposes because people contain many parts, each of which uses the syndrome in a different way, and because people are embedded in complex family and cultural circumstances.

It is also important to note here that Sara's bulimia was oppressive to her and her family, despite the ways that they each used it. Parts of Sara hated her for being unable to control what they saw as a disgustingly gluttonous habit, particularly while living in a family and in a culture where will power ruled supreme. She was so ashamed that she sometimes contemplated suicide. Her parents were wracked with worry, guilt, and embarrassment over the problem. Parts of each of them wanted desperately for Sara to be well, and were willing to do anything to help.

Parallel Levels of Denial. Let me conclude this chapter on cultures and society by drawing one more parallel among system levels. In discussing Sara's family, I have emphasized denial. Her mother had known of her problem for some time, but said she had "just put it out of my mind." Her father's ego was propped up on the shaky belief that he had a seamless, problem-free family. Not only were pain, weakness, failures, and loneliness never discussed; these feelings were not even acknowledged. In this sense, Sara's internal family was a perfect microcosm of her external family. Parts of her denied the existence of her pain and loneliness, and did so successfully for years, until her exiles broke through both her own and her family's denial with the bulimia.

It is no accident that our U.S. society is a perfect macrocosm of Sara's internal and external families. The U.S. government, and parts of many of its citizens, have an amazing ability to deny the pain and suffering that exist in this country. The denial is particularly amazing as the evidence becomes increasingly hard to deny. The incredibly high U.S. murder rate is no longer confined to statistics in the paper or stories on television; murder is happening to people we know. Homeless families are out on the streets. The exiles in cities are erupting at any provocation. Pollution is choking and poisoning children and is affecting the weather and crops. To quote a popular song, "How can we sleep while our beds are burning?"

And yet the United States remains dominated by acquisitive strivers whose (tunnel) vision continues to center on being the best and having the most, with little regard to the worldwide as well as national costs of striving for unlimited growth. As evidence from cultural exiles becomes harder to deny, U.S. society resorts to any number of distractive or numbing firefighter activities, such as patriotic wars on other countries or on drugs, or obsessions with fitness, sporting events, or celebrities' lives.

In a sense, I am proposing a recursive trickle-down theory. Burdens, imbalances, polarizations, and leadership problems funnel from the societal to the familial to the individual levels and back again, creating parallel nested systems that reflect and reinforce one another. There is little evidence of Self-leadership at any level, and we can see the three-group structure (exiles, managers, and firefighters) in operation at each level. Despite the fact that the rest of this book is concerned with helping to balance and harmonize individuals and families, I hope that as therapists we will not limit our activities to these levels and will work to balance and harmonize society as well.

CHAPTER 9

Final Questions and Recommendations

Before ending our exploration of the IFS model, I want to share questions that commonly arise when I teach the model and I want to tie up loose ends.

Can the Model be Used Safely with All Clients?

As I have mentioned in Chapter 1, I use the model in one form or another with every client I treat, because it informs my basic understanding of people; it has become impossible *not* to use it. This does not mean, however, that I use the various techniques described in this book with every client.

The important decision here is whether or not to "go inside" with a client. That is, the techniques of direct access and in-sight open the door to the client's inner world. For some clients this world is scary, fragile, or shameful; they will go to extreme lengths to keep the door closed to themselves and anyone else. When I do not have the proper conditions (described in Chapters 4 and 5) to ensure that we can open the door safely, I will not try to go in. For example, in this age of managed care, many therapist are limited in the number of sessions they can have with many clients (although good managed-care groups know that it pays to provide highly traumatized clients with as many sessions as they need). It is not a good idea for a therapist to open the door to the inner world with a highly polarized client, especially for the purpose of releasing exiles, if the therapist cannot stay with the client at least long enough to help him or her integrate those exiles. I have the same reluctance to expose exiles when a client's external environment is dangerous and intractable, or when a client is in a position in his or her family or job that allows little room for vulnerability. Finally, I will not go inside when, for some reason, I cannot lead with my Self while working with a client. Some people or situations may activate a therapist's parts to such an extent that it is better to remain outside.

Even with time or external constraints or with therapist activation, however, it can be very valuable to help clients understand managers and managerial fears; find that they have Selves; understand firefighters and why these parts are so reactive; find that exiles exist; and see that they can begin to relate to all these parts differently on their own. In other words, even when therapists cannot do the whole job, helping clients know this much can be empowering.

Highly Disturbed Clients?

"In using this model, isn't there a danger of further fragmenting highly disturbed clients?" This question invariably arises when I present the IFS model; the answer to it is yes. But the danger does not come from helping people to view themselves as multiple beings. Highly disturbed clients already know this about themselves and are often relieved to learn that their multiplicity is not a sign of pathology. Their problem lies not in their multiplicity, but in the fact that their parts are highly polarized; they experience little effective leadership inside; and as a result they have little sense of continuity or cohesiveness. When used effectively, the model decreases rather than increases their sense of fragmentation because their extreme, isolated, polarized parts are helped to harmonize, and they feel increasingly integrated and unitary.

The danger of further fragmentation arises from using the model improperly, particularly from not respecting managers and prematurely activating exiles. The ensuing firefighter reactions can be frightening and can trigger further polarization (i.e., fragmentation). In addition, the techniques of direct access and in-sight are powerful and, like anything powerful, can be dangerous if used in an uninformed or careless manner. However, if a therapist follows the guidelines outlined in this book, the techniques are generally safe.

Children and Adolescents?

"Can the model be used with children or adolescents?" Children are often more receptive to the IFS model than adults are. They are closer to the multiplicity phenomenon because they are less thoroughly socialized away from it.   Often children can change more rapidly than adults, because their managers are less interfering and more trusting. Their images are often more fantastic, with parts that look like cartoon characters, animals, monsters, kings, queens, and other such figures. Therapists who use the model with children often have them draw their parts and interact with the drawings. They also use puppets, clay, making up stories, or psychodramatic techniques. All the techniques used in play therapy are adaptable to the model. Similarly, adolescents are often adept with the model, once the therapists can get past the parts of them that worry so much about their image or do not trust adults.

Clients of Varying Sophistication/Education?

"Don't clients need a certain level of psychological sophistication or insight to use this model effectively?" No. People of all levels of intelligence and education are able to access the phenomenon. We have worked successfully with developmentally disabled clients and with many uneducated people from impoverished neighborhoods of Chicago. Most people have an intuition about this process. The task of the therapist is to remain flexible enough to tailor the language that introduces the model to the client so that it is comfortable and understandable. The therapist also must be flexible in accepting the many different ways in which clients do the work.

Indeed, sometimes clients with the most psychological sophistication or most intellectualized style of relating are the most difficult to engage in the model. They are often dominated by protective intellectual managers that have trouble giving up enough control to allow access to other parts. Thus, when a client has trouble using the model, it is rarely because of some kind of deficit; it is usually because of parts that are afraid.

Groups?

"Is the model effective with groups?" I have not run many groups using the model, but many of my colleagues have. They have developed a range of innovative methods that cannot be described in this space. I hope to edit a collection of adaptations that will include group therapy.

Where Do Therapists Commonly Get Stuck?

Every therapist using the IFS model gets stuck. Before I wrote this book, I found that few therapists could learn enough from a workshop to stay with the model beyond their first few stuck points. Instead, they would give it up altogether and retreat to their previous, more comfortable approaches. Even with this book, many therapists will retreat, and that is appropriate. The IFS approach is not a good fit with everyone, and if a therapist does not have at least a modicum of intuition about these ideas, he or she should not try to use the model. For those who want to persevere, however, I present below some common predicaments or mistakes and some suggestions.

Therapist Insecurity

Insecurity is the biggest problem facing beginners. With many clients, the effective use of the IFS model requires that the therapist demonstrate a certain amount of confidence. These clients will not (and should not) open the door to their inner world for therapists who are not sure of what they are doing. The Catch-22 is that most therapists do not feel confident until they have opened the door, found that the model works, and discovered that nothing happens that they cannot handle. For many therapists, the IFS model represents a radical departure from their familiar beliefs and methods. They want proof that the model works before making a major investment in it. Ironically, their skeptical and insecure parts may keep them from getting proof by triggering protective reactions from clients, and consequently they will not be allowed in.

Where supervision or ongoing consultation in the model is not available, the best solution to this dilemma is for the therapist to make a careful choice of the the client with whom he or she begins to use the model. Some clients have not been hurt as severely as others, and consequently have less delicate and protective inner families. Once given the basic principles and techniques, many of these clients know just what to do. They easily enter into exploratory partnerships with their therapists, and often take the lead in these explorations. The insecure beginner, then, is well advised to find such a client/teacher before going inside. After safe explorations of that kind, the beginner's insecure parts may feel safe enough to let him or her start using the model with more polarized clients.

Even experienced IFS therapists will encounter situations where they are puzzled by the work and do not know what to do. This still happens to me on a weekly basis. Gradually, however, an IFS therapist develops trust in his or her Self and in the client's Self. I now have an abiding faith that no matter how confusing or difficult things become while a client and I are exploring the client's inner world, if I lead with my Self and ask my client's Self for help, eventually we will prevail. Until a therapist acquires this faith, it will be difficult to overcome many of the apparently insurmountable obstacles that arise along the path. This faith is probably the most important quality an experienced IFS supervisor can bring to the beginner.

The other necessary ability that faith in one's Self-leadership provides is flexibility. The more a therapist can enter a client's inner system without a preset and fixed agenda, but rather with the attitude that if necessary he or she will go wherever the client's system leads, the better. So many unforeseen events occur on these journeys that this flexible attitude is crucial. Also, clients' parts relax when they sense such flexibility in their therapists, and their own ability to be in control. This requires that therapists, however, give up the security that comes from being in control themselves—from being able to predict just what is going to happen and how it will be handled. Again, it requires trust in a therapist's Self. In some sections of this book, procedures have been laid out in formulaic fashion; these are meant as general guidelines, not rigid rules that might impair flexibility.

The only caveat regarding this flexible attitude is not to forget that as a client approaches certain feared thresholds, parts often emerge that want to distract and lead wild goose chases. If the therapist senses this, he or she should ask the client's Self whether this seems to be the case, and, if so, should work with the distractings parts' fears.

A related point is that although I have stressed the delicacy of this work with severely polarized and hurt clients, it is also true that a therapist can recover from mistakes if there is a connection between the therapist's and the client's Selves. Mistakes can produce extreme reactions, but if the therapist and client can remain connected through these ecological crises, the trust in their relationship can be strengthened. Generally, the fearful or protective parts of the therapist are what turn a mistake into a dangerous situation. In that sense, to borrow a phrase, the only thing a therapist has to fear is fear itself. For example, when a therapist who maintains Self-leadership inadvertently activates an exile prematurely, he or she can calm the exile and the managers, even in the face of their extreme reactions. If a fearful or protective part of the therapist takes over, however, the client will feel abandoned, and the client's parts will escalate their reactions.

The point is that it is not the nature of the work that makes it dangerous, but the potential for escalations among parts of client and therapist. If the therapist can maintain Self-leadership—can remain the "I in the storm"—the potential for escalation is greatly reduced and mistakes can be overcome. I know this is true, because I have made and continue to make many, many mistakes. Therapists should work with the parts of them that fear mistakes, instead of letting such parts constrain their work.

Therapist Responsibility

Many beginners are insecure because they are afraid to trust their *clients'* Selves. They believe that as therapists, they have the primary responsibility to create change. As a result, they are highly directive and stimulate power struggles with clients' parts. They make many interpretations and leap to conclusions. They expose exiles too quickly and disregard feedback from managers. In other words, their therapy is dominated by their striving, controlling, or caretaking parts. They encounter more resistance than therapists who trusts their clients' Selves because clients' managers do not like to be told what to do or how they think or feel. As with so many things in life, the harder one tries, the more one fails.

To counter this tendency, the beginner is encouraged to watch his or her language. There are many instances where, instead of telling a client what to do with a part, the therapist can ask the client what he or she thinks should happen. Many beginners do not make this shift from directive to inquisitive language as soon as they could. Once a client's Self is somewhat differentiated, he or she often knows how to help her parts. The therapist's role becomes that of helping the client remain differentiated and supporting his or her intuition. If the therapist remains in the directive or interpretive position, client differentiation is impeded, so the therapist should periodically shift to the inquisitive style and see how the client responds. Beginning IFS therapists are frequently amazed at how much their clients already know when asked these questions.

Lack of Parts Detection

Probably the most common mistake beginners make is assuming they are talking to a client's Self when they are talking to a part. For example, at one time or another clients may seem confused; say that they cannot do something; no longer see their parts; criticize the model or the therapist; intellectualize about their problems or their inner work; or launch lengthy, detailed discussions about their week. Sometimes these issues are legitimate and are important to address. At other times, however, parts are interfering in subtle, deceptive ways. People have parts that can sound quite reasonable and can present their extreme or distracting positions in convincing ways.

A beginning therapist often takes the bait and either believes what a part is saying or enters into an argument with it (thus contributing to its distractive purpose). An experienced IFS therapist, in contrast, develops a highly sensitive "parts detector." That is, through cues such as tone of voice and shift in posture, in addition to the extremeness of the content, the experienced therapist develops a sense for when a person is and is not leading with the Self. When the therapist suspects the work of a subtle part, he or she asks for the client's Self to see whether such a part is there, rather than dealing with the part directly. Once the part has been detected, the therapist can talk to it directly or can have the client's Self interact with it through in-sight.

I prefer not to argue with parts when they are extreme and trying to create a distraction or are otherwise protecting other parts. Sometimes this is very difficult, because parts of me are easily lured into arguments, and certain clients seem to have a knack for activating them. Rather than arguing, a therapist can reassure the client's part that its interference is not necessary, and/or ask why the part is interfering. Arguing with parts usually only makes them more extreme and gives them more power. There is an old Chinese adage: "Never wrestle with a swine, because you both get filthy and the swine enjoys it." With apologies for the porcine analogy, I have learned the hard way not to wrestle with certain parts.

Similarly, there are times when a beginning therapist will believe that the person's Self is working with his or her parts when in fact a "Self surrogate" is doing this for the Self. For people who can see their inner worlds clearly, there is an easy way to check whether this is the case. If the person can *see* himself or herself doing the work—for example, entering the room with a part and conversing with it—then the Self is not doing it. Instead, the Self is watching two parts interact. With in-sight, the Self is invisible; the Self is the seat of consciousness, the place from which a person sees and interacts with his or her parts. Again, a therapist who suspects that a part is leading for a client's Self should ask the Self to find the part and reassure it that the Self can do it.

Not Fully Exploring a Part's Constraints

Many beginners confuse a part with its role. They judge the book by its cover. They believe the extreme things that parts say about themselves, and come to see the parts as defective, incorrigible, or deliberately destructive. Even for experienced IFS therapists, some parts persistently interfere to the point that such conclusions are hard to resist. When this happens, the therapists' parts are easily engaged in power struggles with the clients' parts. The therapists lose the conviction that no part likes its extreme role and would not remain in it if not for a variety of constraints.

This is particularly true in a case where the therapist has tried to understand and help a part with a number of constraints, and still the part maintains its extremeness. Despite this frustration, it always pays off to remain patient and hold fast to the belief that there remains a constraint that has not yet been released. Sometimes a therapist will have depolarized, retrieved, and unburdened a part, only finally to discover a key constraining part that has been hiding behind the scenes. Or there is a person or situation in the client's external life that the client has been afraid to mention and that chronically activates the part. Or the culprit may be a part of the therapist lurking around, of which the therapist is unaware.

Many therapists become impatient when, after working with managers and firefighters, they seem to be on the brink of meeting exiles, and yet the managers and firefighters continue their evasive tactics. For many clients, exposing their exiles is a terrifying proposition. Their managers will not open the door until they are certain it is safe. Even when a therapist believes every managerial fear has been addressed, there are often undisclosed fears. The most common of these have to do with activating scary firefighters (such as those urging suicide, rage, or sexual acting out) or disconnection from external family members. Also, releasing the exiles may force managers to confront their own exiled feelings, so these managers first need a solid relationship with the therapist. The therapist's impatience or frustration will always prolong these delays that commonly precede meeting exiles. Indeed, this impatience may be the primary hidden constraint that managers are afraid to mention.

Mark Twain once said, "Habit is habit, and not to be thrown down the stairs, but coaxed down one step at a time." Managers are in the habit of being fearful and cautious; they should be coaxed down from their protective perch one step at a time.

Not Exploring or Working with a Client's External Context

The IFS model opens the door to a fascinating and powerful inner world. Many beginners become so intrigued with this internal aspect of the model that they ignore the impact of and resources in the clients' families or other external contexts. This is particularly true for therapists whose training has been in individual treatment and who have not been taught to appreciate or work with external systems. But even family therapists can succumb to the temptation to go inside with clients and close the door on the storms raging outside. I have to fight this temptation with many clients, and I have a PhD in family therapy.

A therapist can overestimate the ability of a client to transcend the constraints of his or her family or other external circumstances by doing internal work. When brainstorming with the client about whom to involve in the treatment, the therapist must take care not to collude with parts of the client that want to deny external constraints. If the client wants to keep a person out of the therapy room or does not want to talk about an external relationship, it is often worth talking to the parts making the request, in order to gauge the purity of their motives.

The larger point here is that although it is tempting to ignore external constraints, it can also be costly. IFS therapy is shorter, safer, and more effective when constraints and resources of *all* levels are considered.

Therapists who are disinclined by training or by nature to work with external people should pursue family therapy training, and should also work with their parts that fear the intensity of family therapy.

Therapist Parts

All the ways therapists get stuck that I have described above are related to the interference of therapist parts. Chapters 4 and 7 have detailed other common problems caused by therapist parts. I cannot emphasize enough the importance of IFS therapists' being aware at least of those of their parts that may interfere in therapy. The injunction to "Know thyself" changes to "Know thy parts." I strongly encourage trainees to work with their parts constantly. This does not necessarily mean finding an IFS therapist to work with; many people can do a great deal of work on their own and only need a therapist when they get stuck. Also, many therapists who do not know the IFS model are sensitive and competent people who can provide a safe and stimulating environment in which such explorations can take place.

I also encourage trainees to work with their parts before, during, and after sessions when they reach impasses or sessions that are particularly activating. The Self-confidence technique described in Chapter 7 is useful in this struggle. The therapist can put a particularly activating client in a room in his or her mind and gather together the parts that react to the client. By asking these parts what upsets them and why, and then asking for them not to interfere, the therapist can grow.

In addition, a therapist can encourage his or her clients to use their own parts detectors—to let the therapist know when they think he or she is not totally there. Not only does this help the therapist, but clients feel empowered and safe when they know they can have some effect on the way the therapist relates to them.

How Can a Therapist Keep Going?

How can a beginner stay with the IFS model, despite repeatedly getting stuck in these many morasses? As I have implied, it helps to have access to an experienced consultant. In Chicago, there are many IFS consultation groups; these groups meet at intervals that vary from twice a month to four times per year. In a number of other communities, particularly in the Midwest, therapists have organized peer consultation groups around the model. There are also other models that respect the multiplicity phenomenon and can provide training or consultation. In general, then, it helps a great deal to find other therapists with whom to share this fascinating journey.

Finally, it helps to remember that therapists' caseloads are full of excellent teachers. Among Eastern religions, there is an adage: "When the student is ready, the teacher will be there." For IFS therapists, the teachers are already there, so the goal is to get ready.

Conclusion

This book captures the IFS model at a single point in its development, the way a snapshot captures a child who will continue to change dramatically in the years to come. The model is in constant motion. Concepts and techniques have been repeatedly added and refined, as well as dropped, since the early years. I will be surprised and disappointed if aspects of this book are not outdated within 2 years. I believe, however, that the basic assumptions and methods will hold up well over time.

The main constraints to the model's early evolution have been my own preconceptions and biases—in other words, my parts. As my relationship with my parts improves, the pace of evolution increases, because I am less attached to my preconceptions and more open to my clients' lessons. In addition, the number of other therapists who know the model well enough to contribute has reached critical mass. These others are expanding the model, particularly in the area of technique, in ways that I never imagined. I am heartened and delighted by these contributions and look forward to seeing where they lead. I firmly believe that the current IFS model only scratches the surface of what is possible if we pursue this path.

APPENDIX A

Summary Outline for Working with Individuals

Because the methods described in Chapters 4 and 5 are varied and complex, an outline for the IFS approach to individuals is provided below. Like everything about the IFS model, however, this outline should not be adhered to rigidly; it represents only one of many ways in which IFS therapy with individuals can be sequenced.

I. Introducing the model.
   A. Client describes problem, and therapist feeds back what client says using the language of parts.
   B. Therapist introduces basic concepts of model.
      1. Everyone has parts and Self.
      2. Goal: To get client's parts to get along with one another and help client's Self.
      3. This can be done safely, with respect for client's pace.
   C. Therapist asks whether client is interested in working this way.
      1. If no, therapist explores client's fears and backs off if necessary, with option of asking again later after more trust is developed.
      2. If yes, therapist proceeds to II.

II. Getting to know the territory.
   A. Therapist asks client to describe parts that he or she is aware of, and asks questions about client's relationship with each part and their relationships with one another. (Experienced IFS therapists can sometimes skip this step.)
   B. Therapist and client discuss client's external context, with an eye toward the following:
      1. People or situations that are activating client's parts.

      2. People or situations that might react negatively to changes in client resulting from the work.

  C. Therapist and client assess ability to proceed internally, given client's external context.

      1. If external context is too activating or dangerous, therapist and client work to change it first; this may entail bringing in family members (see Chapter 7).

      2. If there is enough room in external context to do some internal work, therapist and client proceed to III, while carefully watching external context and working with it as needed.

III. Entering client's internal family.

  A. Therapist addresses managers first.

      1. Therapist asks client about any parts that worry about going inside.

      2. Therapist asks client about parts that are even slightly uncomfortable about therapist or about therapist–client relationship.

  B. Therapist discusses common manager concerns as much as seems necessary by doing one of the following:

      1. Talking to client while managers listen.

      2. Directly accessing managers.

      3. Having Self talk to managers through in-sight.

  C. Common manager concerns include the following:

      1. Exiles cannot change.

      2. Exiles will take over if given any access.

      3. Therapist will reject or abandon client for having exiles.

      4. Client's external context is not safe.

      5. Going in will trigger dangerous firefighters.

  D. Therapist and managers discuss concerns until some level of permission to proceed is received.

  E. Therapist makes rough guess as to client's level of Self-differentiation and trust, based on these discussions.

      1. If perceived level of differentiation is high, then therapist can skip many of the precautionary steps in IV, until proven wrong.

      2. If perceived level is low, therapist proceeds slowly and follows IV carefully.

IV. Depolarizing parts and differentiating Self.

  A. Therapist asks client which part he or she would like to start with.

      1. If client selects what is likely to be an exile (e.g., "my sad part"), therapist asks to talk first with parts that might be afraid for client to work with exile, but reassures exile that it will eventually be addressed.

      2. If client selects a firefighter (e.g., "the part that makes me drink"), direct access is not recommended until managers have been con-

sulted; therapist uses in-sight room technique, ensuring initially that part is safely secured in room.

3. If client selects a manager (e.g., "my critical part"), therapist can use direct access or in-sight.

B. Once a part is selected (let's call it part *A*), therapist checks how differentiated client's Self is relative to part *A*.

1. Therapist asks how client feels toward part *A*.

2. If response is along the lines of compassion, curiosity, or acceptance, therapist skips to V.

2. If response is anything besides compassion, curiosity, or acceptance, therapist asks client to find and separate from parts that are polarized with or activated by part *A* and are interfering.

3. If polarized parts will separate and Self seems differentiated enough to proceed, therapist and client's Self skip to V.

C. When relationship between part *A* and other parts is polarized to the point that parts refuse to differentiate from Self, the following occurs:

1. Therapist or client's Self accesses each part involved in the polarization and discusses fears or anger.

2. If, after discussion, polarized parts agree to separate from Self when it talks to part *A*, therapist and Self skip to V.

3. If polarized parts continue to refuse to separate, work takes place with each of them first, as in V, and then returns later to part A.

V. Identifying constraints impinging on an individual part.

A. If client's Self is somewhat differentiated, then Self works with part *A*.

1. If part *A* is a manager or firefighter, therapist has Self ask part questions designed to identify constraints and give hope:

a. Why it does it do what it does?

b. What does it really want for the person, beneath its extreme intention statements?

c. What is it afraid will happen if it leaves its extreme role? Which other part(s) is it polarized with or protecting?

d. What role would it like if it no longer had to play this one? What does it need from Self or therapist to be able to make the shift to the new role?

e. What burdens does it carry, and where it is stuck in the past (where did it get these burdens)?

2. If part *A* is an exile, blending is a concern; thus, before Self gets close to part, Self and therapist do the following:

a. Self asks part to try to contain its feelings as Self approaches it.

b. If part agrees, therapist tells Self to get as close to part as possible without being overwhelmed by its feelings.

c. If exile cannot contain its feelings, such that Self is overwhelmed, therapist asks Self to back away and asks again for part to try not to blend.

    d. If part is still unable to contain feelings, therapist talks to part directly, comforting it and reassuring that it will be released from exile and taken care of eventually.

    e. If part is able to contain blending, Self works with exile, particularly in regard to retrieving it from the past and unburdening it.

B. If client's parts will not differentiate from Self or if part A cannot contain blending, therapist directly accesses part A and identifies its constraints as described above.

VI. Releasing constraints impinging on an individual part.

  A. Depolarizing with another part.

    1. Self meets with each part individually and asks both if they are willing to face each other.

    2. If so, Self has polarized parts interact until they see each other differently and construct a new relationship.

  B. Releasing part A from having to protect other parts.

    1. Self finds parts that A protects and works with them so that they are not so vulnerable and in need of protection.

    2. Self helps A find and unload any burdens of protectiveness (see Unburdening a part, below).

  C. Retrieving part from where it is stuck in the past.

    1. Self gets close to part without blending and gains part's confidence.

    2. Self checks with managers about any fears they have regarding going back (particularly fears of triggering rageful, suicidal, or other scary firefighters).

    3. Self deals with those firefighters first (if necessary).

    4. Therapist checks to be sure Self is differentiated and feels ready to handle retrieval.

    5. Self asks part to show where it is stuck in the past.

    6. Part shows Self a scene.

    7. Self tells part to show as much as it needs to to be able to leave, and Self waits until part has shown all.

    8. Self enters scene and is there in the way the person needed someone to be there when it happened (i.e., does whatever necessary to help part).

    9. Self asks part whether there is anything it wants done before it is ready to leave and come into the present with Self, and then Self and part do those things.

   10. Self and part come into the present and find a place for part to stay that is safe and comfortable (if no place in present feels safe, this could be an imaginary place or a place in the past that was safe).

11. Self asks for volunteers among parts to stay with and care for retrieved part, and then evaluates the fit with whatever parts volunteer.
12. Self agrees on a schedule to visit retrieved part.
13. Self checks with managers to see which ones are upset by retrieval and what they need not to sabotage it.

D. Unburdening a part.
   1. Self asks part whether it knows that the extreme feeling or belief (burden) is not intrinsic to itself but was put on or in it.
   2. If answer is no, Self helps part find where it got the burden by doing a retrieval (return to C above), in which part can see that the burden was given to it.
   3. Once part knows burden was put on it, Self asks part to find the burden either in or on it.
   4. Part finds burden (part can often see something that symbolizes it), and Self helps part remove it.
   5. Self and part decide what to do with or where to leave burden so that part no longer has to carry it.
   6. Self checks with other parts to see whether any of them are upset about unburdening, and addresses their feelings.

E. Inviting lost parts to return.
   1. Self asks unburdened and retrieved part to invite any parts of it (essentially subparts) that left during traumatic episodes to return to its body.
   2. Sometimes nothing happens. Other times Self can see many subparts returning.

F. Finding a new role for part.
   1. After being released from some or all of the constraints above, some parts will immediately know the new role they prefer; other parts, however, will have no idea what to do.
   2. Self discusses with part A a variety of alternatives, considering the part's strengths, talents, and goals.
   3. Part A makes ultimate decision on new role.
   4. Part A, in new role, is introduced to other parts.

G. Additional guidelines.
   1. If part will not differentiate from client's Self sufficiently, then steps A–D above can be done through direct access, with the therapist temporarily in the role of Self. (With some clients, this becomes the primary method.)
   2. Whenever there is any problem throughout steps A–D, it should be assumed to be caused by an interfering part. Therapist or client's Self should try to get it to separate (interfering part may be in therapist).

3. Parts can be put in rooms to assist in keeping them separated.
4. Parts should never be coerced into compliance; if they refuse to comply, work should be done with their fears until they are ready.
5. Exiles are not the only parts that carry burdens or are stuck in the past; often, managers and firefighters do/are too, but try to hide from these feelings behind their roles.

VII. Harmonizing the internal family.
   A. Convening and assessing the internal family.
      1. As key polarizations are resolved and parts become less extreme, client's Self can ask for them all to come together. (When internal system is less polarized to begin with, the internal family can meet together from the start.)
      2. Self examines how the group assembles, and often can sense where polarizations remain.
      3. Self asks group about parts or internal relationships that remain extreme.
   B. Depolarizing the internal family.
      1. Self has polarized parts come forward from the group, one pair at a time, and becomes their therapist as they discuss their issues.
      2. After each pair resolves issues and makes agreements, Self asks group for feedback.
   C. Synchronizing new roles.
      1. As parts depolarize and adopt new roles, Self meets with the group to help all members find ways to fit new roles together well.
   D. Group decision making.
      1. As decisions emerge in the person's life, Self assembles parts for internal board meetings in which the group discusses the decision.
      2. Self listens to this discussion and then makes the decision.
      3. Self takes care of those parts that lost out in the decision, and tries to maintain balance such that no part or group of parts always loses.
   E. Mobilizing the group for a specific task.
      1. Self meets with group of parts and describes the task or crisis at hand.
      2. Parts discuss which of them should be involved and how they should work together until a plan is achieved.

Ultimately, this process can result in a harmonious internal family whose members work and play together with respect and cooperation, and trust the leadership of the Self. The time it takes to achieve this end can vary greatly, depending largely on how polarized and distrusting the person's internal and external systems are at the outset, and how much Self-leadership the therapist can maintain.

APPENDIX B

Glossary of Concepts

Balance: A state in which members at the same level of a human system have equitable access to the responsibilities, resources, and influence they need.

Blending: When the feelings and beliefs of one part merge with another part or the Self.

Burdens: Extreme ideas or feelings that are carried by parts and govern their lives. Burdens are left on or in parts from exposure to an external person or event.

Constraining environment: A human system's environment characterized by imbalance, polarizations, enmeshments, and problematic leadership. Constraining environments impose burdens on the systems within them.

Effective leadership: Leadership characterized by compassion, fairness, vision, and nurturance.

Enmeshment: A state in which two members (or two groups) in a system become highly interdependent, to the point where both parties' access to their Selves is constrained because their parts are so reactive to one another.

Exiles: Parts that are sequestered within a system, for their own protection or for the protection of the system from them.

Feedback: Information received by a system from its environment.

Feedwithin: Information communicated among members of a system.

Firefighters: Parts that go into action after the exiles have been activated, to calm the exiles or distract the system from them (dissociation).

Harmony: A state in which the members of a human system relate collaboratively, with effective communication, mutual caring, and a sense of connection.

Imbalance: A state in which one member (or a group) has more or less access to responsibilities, influence, and resources.

Managers: Parts that try to run a system in ways that minimize the activation (upset) of the exiles.

Multiplicity paradigm: The recognition that the human mind is not unitary, but instead is naturally subdivided into a multitude of subpersonalities.

Parts: The term used in IFS for a person's subpersonalities. Parts are best considered internal people of different ages, talents, and temperaments.

Polarization: A state in which two members (or two groups) in a system relate in opposition to or in competition with each other, to the point where each party's access to the Self is constrained by fear that the other party will win or take over.

Problematic leadership: A state in which leaders of a system have abdicated, are biased, are polarized with each other, or have been discredited.

Self: The core of a person, which contains leadership qualities such as compassion, perspective, curiosity, and confidence. The Self is best equipped to lead the internal family.

Sustaining environment: A human system's environment characterized by balance, harmony, and effective leadership.

APPENDIX C

Bibliography of Models of Multiplicity

Assagioli, R. (1973). *The act of will*. New York: Penguin Books.

Assagioli, R. (1975). *Psychosynthesis: A manual of principles and techniques*. London: Turnstone Press. (Original work published 1965)

Bandler, J., & Grinder, R. (1982). *Reframing*. Moab, UT: Real People Press.

Beahrs, J. O. (1982). *Unity and multiplicity*. New York: Brunner/Mazel.

Berne, E. (1961). *Transactional analysis in psychotherapy*. New York: Grove Press.

Berne, E. (1972). *What do you say after you say hello?* New York: Grove Press.

Bliss, E. L. (1986). *Multiple personality, allied disorders, and hypnosis*. New York: Oxford University Press.

Breunlin, D., Schwartz, R. C., & Mac Kune-Karrer, B. (1992). *Metaframeworks: Transcending the models of family therapy*. San Francisco: Jossey-Bass.

Csikszentmihalyi, M. (1990). *Flow: The psychology of optimal experience*. New York: Harper & Row.

Federn, P. (1952). *Ego psychology and the psychoses*. New York: Basic Books.

Ferrucci, P. (1982). *What we may be*. Los Angeles: J. P. Tarcher.

Freud, S. (1961). The ego and the id. In J. Strachey (Ed. and Trans.), *The standard edition of the complete psychological works of Sigmund Freud* (Vol. 19). London: Hogarth Press. (Original work published 1923)

Freud, S. (1964). Splitting of the ego in the process of defence. In J. Strachey (Ed. and Trans.), *The standard edition of the complete psychological works of Sigmund Freud* (Vol. 23). London: Hogarth Press. (Original work published 1940)

Gazzaniga, M. (1985). *The social brain*. New York: Basic Books.

Goulding, R., & Schwartz, R. C. (in press). *Mosaic mind: Empowering the tormented selves of child abuse survivors*. New York: W. W. Norton.

Hannah, B. (1981). *Encounters with the soul: Active imagination as developed by C. G. Jung*. Boston: Sigo Press.

Harner, M. (1990). *The way of the shaman*. San Francisco: HarperCollins.

Hesse, H. (1975). *Treatise on the Steppenwolf* (J. Bradac, Trans.). London: Wildwood House. (Original work published 1927)

Hillman, J. (1975). *Re-visioning psychology*. New York: Harper & Row.

Hofstadter, D. (1986). *Metamagical themas*. New York: Bantam Books.

Ingerman, S. (1991). *Soul retrieval: Mending the fragmented self*. San Francisco: HarperCollins.

Johnson, R. (1986). *Inner work: Using dreams and active imagination for personal growth*. San Francisco: Harper & Row.

Jung, C. G. (1956). *Two essays on analytical psychology*. Cleveland, OH: Meridian.

Jung, C. G. (1962). *Memories, dreams, reflections* (A. Jaffè, Ed.; R. Winston & C. Winston, Trans.). New York: Pantheon Books.

Jung, C. G. (1969). *The collected works of C. G. Jung (2nd ed.): Vol. 8, Part I. The structure and dynamics of the psyche* (H. Read, M. Fordham, & G. Adler, Eds.; R. F. C. Hull, Trans.). Princeton, NJ: Princeton University Press.

Jung, C. G. (1971). *The collected works of C. G. Jung (2nd ed.): Vol. 9, Part I. The archetypes and the collective unconscious* (H. Read, M. Fordham, & G. Adler, Eds.; R. F. C. Hull, Trans.). Princeton, NJ: Princeton University Press.

Markus, H., & Nurius, P. (1987). Possible selves: The interface between motivation and the self-concept. In K. Yardley & T. Honess (Eds.), *Self and identity: Psychosocial perspectives*. Chichester, England: Wiley.

Miller, A. (1981). *The drama of the gifted child*. New York: Basic Books.

Minsky, M. (1986). *The society of mind*. New York: Simon & Schuster.

Napier, N. (1990). *Recreating your self: Help for adult children of dysfuntional families*. New York: W. W. Norton.

Napier, N. (1993). *Getting through the day: Strategies for adults hurt as children*. New York: W. W. Norton.

O'Connor, E. (1971). *Our many selves: A handbook for self discovery*. New York: Harper & Row.

Ornstein, R. (1986). *Multiminds: A new way to look at human behavior*. Boston: Houghton Mifflin.

Perls, F. (1969). *Gestalt therapy verbatim*. Moab, UT: Real People Press.

Putnam, F. W. (1989). *Diagnosis and treatment of multiple personality disorder*. New York: Guilford Press.

Redfern, J. (1985). *My self, my many selves*. London: Academic Press.

Rowan, J. (1990). *Subpersonalities: The people inside us*. London: Routledge.

Satir, V. (1978). *Your many faces*. Berkeley, CA: Celestial Arts.

Satir, V., & Baldwin, M. (1983). *Satir step by step*. Palo Alto, CA: Science & Behavior Books.

Schwartz, R. C. (1987). Our multiple selves. *Family Therapy Networker, 11*, 25–31, 80–83.

Schwartz, R. C. (1988). Know thy selves. *Family Therapy Networker, 12*, 21–29.

Schwartz, R. C. (1992). Rescuing the exiles. *Family Therapy Networker, 16*, 33–37, 75.

Schwartz, R. C. (1993, Winter). Constructionism, sex abuse, and the self. *American Family Therapy Academy Newsletter*, pp. 6–10.

Sliker, G. (1992). *Multiple mind*. Boston: Shambala Press.

Stone, H., & Stone, S. (1993). *Embracing your inner critic*. San Francisco: HarperCollins.

Stone, H., & Winkelman, S. (1985). *Embracing ourselves*. Marina del Rey, CA: Devross.

Stone, H., & Winkelman, S. (1989). *Embracing each other*. San Rafael, CA: New World Library.

Varela, F., Thompson, E., & Rosch, E. (1991). *The embodied mind*. Cambridge, MA: MIT Press.

Watanabe, S. (1986). Cast of characters work: Systematically exploring the naturally organized personality. *Contemporary Family Therapy, 8*, 75–83.

Watkins, J. (1978). *The therapeutic self*. New York: Human Sciences Press.

Watkins, J., & Johnson, R. J. (1982). *We, the divided self*. New York: Irvington.

Watkins, J., & Watkins, H. (1979). Ego states and hidden observers. *Journal of Altered States of Consciousness, 5*, 3–18.

Watkins, J., & Watkin, H. (1982). Ego state therapy. In L. E. Abt & I. R. Stuart (Eds.). *The newer therapies: A sourcebook*. New York: Van Nostrand Reinhold.

Watkins, M. (1986). *Invisible guests: The development of imaginal dialogues*. Hillsdale, NJ: Analytic Press.

Wright, R. (1986, March–April). A better mental model. *The Sciences*, pp. 26–28.

References

Anderson, C. (1982). The community connection: The impact of social networks on family and individual functioning. In F. Walsh (Ed.), *Normal Family Processes*. New York: Guilford Press.

Assagioli, R. (1973). *The act of will*. New York: Penguin Books.

Assagioli, R. (1975). *Psychosynthesis: A manual of principles and techniques*. London: Turnstone Press. (Original work published 1965)

Bandler, J., & Grinder, R. (1982). *Reframing*. Moab, UT: Real People Press.

Bateson, G., & Jackson, D. (1964). Some varieties of pathogenic organization. *Disorders of Communication, 42*, 270–283.

Bateson, G. (1970). A systems approach. *International Journal of Psychiatry, 9*, 242–244.

Beahrs, J. O. (1982). *Unity and multiplicity*. New York: Brunner/Mazel.

Bellah, R. N., Madsen, R., Sullivan, W. M., Swidler, A., & Tipton, S. M. (1985). *Habits of the heart: Individualism and commitment in American life*. New York: Harper & Row.

Berne, E. (1961). *Transactional analysis in psychotherapy*. New York: Grove Press.

Berne, E. (1972). *What do you say after you say hello?* New York: Grove Press.

Bliss, E. L. (1986). *Multiple personality, allied disorders, and hypnosis*. New York: Oxford University Press.

Bowen, M. (1978). *Family therapy in clinical practice*. New York: Jason Aronson.

Breunlin, D., Schwartz, R. C., & Mac Kune-Karrer, B. (1992). *Metaframeworks: Transcending the models of family therapy*. San Francisco: Jossey-Bass.

Carter, E., & McGoldrick, M. (Eds.). (1989). *The changing family life cycle: A framework for family therapy* (2nd ed.). Needham Heights, MA: Allyn & Bacon.

Cecchin, G. (1987). Hypothesizing, circularity, and neutrality revisited: An invitation to curiosity. *Family Process, 26*, 405–413.

Cixous, H. (1974). The character of "character." *New Literary History, 5*, 383–402.

The Compact Edition of the Oxford English Dictionary. (1971). New York: Oxford University Press.

Cook, T. (1990). *Night secrets*. New York: G. P. Putnam's Sons.

Csikszentmihalyi, M. (1990). *Flow: The psychology of optimal experience*. New York: Harper & Row.

Dryden, W., & Golden, W. (Eds.). (1986). *Cognitive–behavioral approaches to psychotherapy*. London: Harper & Row.

Fagan, J., & Sheppard, I. (Eds.). (1970). *Gestalt therapy now*. Palo Alto, CA: Science & Behavior Books.

Fairbairn, W. R. (1952). *An object relations theory of the personality*. London: Tavistock.

Fairburn, C. G., Hay, P. J., & Welch, S. L. (1993). Binge eating and bulimia nervosa: Distribution and determinants. In C. G. Fairburn & G. T. Wilson (Eds.), *Binge eating*. New York: Guilford Press.

Fairburn, C. G., Marcus, M. D., & Wilson, J. (1993). Cognitive–behavioral therapy for binge eating and bulimia nervosa: A comprehensive treatment manual. In C. G. Fairburn & G. T. Wilson (Eds.), *Binge eating*. New York: Guilford Press.

Falicov, C. (Ed.). (1983). *Cultural perspectives in family therapy*. Rockville, MD: Aspen.

Falicov, C., & Brudner-White, L. (1983). The shifting family triangle: The issue of cultural and contextual relativity. In C. Falicov (Ed.), *Cultural perspectives in family therapy*. Rockville, MD: Aspen.

Ferrucci, P. (1982). *What we may be*. Los Angeles: J.P. Tarcher.

Freud, S. (1961). The ego and the id. In J. Strachey (Ed. and Trans.), *The standard edition of the complete psychological works of Sigmund Freud* (Vol. 19). London: Hogarth Press. (Original work published 1923)

Gazzaniga, M. (1985). *The social brain*. New York: Basic Books.

Gitlin, T. (1983). *Inside prime time*. New York: Pantheon.

Goulding, R., & Schwartz, R. C. (in press). *Mosaic mind: Empowering the tormented selves of child abuse survivors*. New York: W. W. Norton.

Gunthrip, H. (1971). *Psychoanalytic theory, therapy and the self*. New York: Basic Books.

Haley, J. (1976). *Problem-solving therapy*. San Francisco: Jossey-Bass.

Haley, J. (1980). *Leaving home*. New York: McGraw-Hill.

Hannah, B. (1981). *Encounters with the soul: Active imagination as developed by C. G. Jung*. Boston: Sigo Press.

Harding, S. (1986). *The science question in feminism*. Ithaca, NY: Cornell University Press.

Hareven, T. (1982). American families in transition: Historical perspectives on change. In F. Walsh (Ed.), *Normal family processes*. New York: Guilford Press.

Harner, M. (1990). *The way of the Shaman*. San Francisco: HarperCollins.

Herman, J. (1992). *Trauma and recovery*. New York: Basic Books.

Hesse, H. (1975). *Treatise on the Steppenwolf* (J. Bradac, Trans.). London: Wildwood House. (Original work published 1927)

Hilgard, E. R. (1977). The problem of divided consciousness: A neodissociation interpretation. *Annals of the New York Academy of Sciences, 296,* 48–59.

Hilgard, E. R. (1979). Divided consciousness in hypnosis: The implications of the hidden observer. In E. Fromm & K. E. Shor (Eds.), *Hypnosis: Developments in research and new perspectives* (2nd ed.). New York: Aldine.

Hillman, J. (1975). *Re-visioning psychology*. New York: Harper & Row.

Hofstadter, D. (1986). *Metamagical themas*. New York: Bantam Books.

Ingerman, S. (1991). *Soul retrieval: Mending the fragmented self.* San Francisco: HarperCollins.

Johnson, C. (1991) *Psychodynamic treatment of anorexia nervosa and bulimia.* New York: Guilford Press.

Johnson, R. (1986). *Inner work: Using dreams and active imagination for personal growth.* San Francisco: Harper & Row.

Jung, C. G. (1956). *Two essays on analytical psychology.* New York: Meridian.

Jung, C. G. (1963). *Memories, dreams, reflections* (A. Jaffè, Ed.; R. Winston & C. Winston, Trans.). New York: Pantheon Books.

Jung, C. G. (1968). *Analytical psychology: Its theory and practice–The Tavistock lectures.* London: Routledge and Kegan Paul. (Original work published 1935)

Jung, C. G. (1968). *The collected works of C. G. Jung (2nd ed.): Vol. 9, Part I. The archetypes and the collective unconscious* (H. Read, M. Fordham, & G. Adler, Eds.; R. F. C. Hull, Trans.). Princeton, NJ: Princeton University Press.

Jung, C. G. (1969). *The collected works of C. G. Jung (2nd ed.): Vol. 8. The structure and dynamics of the psyche* (H. Read, M. Fordham, & G. Adler, Eds.; R. F. C. Hull, Trans.). Princeton, NJ: Princeton University Press.

Kernberg, O. (1976). *Object relations theory and clinical psychoanalysis.* New York: Jason Aronson.

Kerr, M., & Bowen, M. (1988). *Family evaluation.* New York: Norton.

Klein, M. (1948). *Contributions to psychoanalysis.* London: Hogarth Press.

Kluft, R. P. (Ed.). (1985). *Childhood antecedents of multiple personality disorder.* Washington, DC: American Psychiatric Press.

Kohut, H. (1971). *The Analysis of the self.* New York: International Universities Press.

Kohut, H. (1977). *The restoration of the self.* New York: International Universities Press.

Madanes, C. (1981). *Strategic family therapy.* San Francisco: Jossey-Bass.

Markus, H., & Nurius, P. (1987). Possible selves: The interface between motivation and the self-concept. In K. Yardley & T. Honess (Eds.), *Self and identity: Psychosocial perspectives.* Chichester, England: Wiley.

McGoldrick, M., Pearce, J., & Giordano, J. (Eds.). (1982). *Ethnicity and family therapy.* New York: Guilford Press.

Miller, A. (1981). *The drama of the gifted child.* New York: Basic Books.

Minsky, M. (1986). *The society of mind.* New York: Simon & Schuster.

Mintz, N., & Schwartz, D. (1964). Urban ecology and psychosis. *International Journal of Social Psychiatry, 10,* 101–118.

Minuchin, S. (1974). *Families and family therapy.* Cambridge, MA: Harvard University Press.

Minuchin, S., & Fishman, H. C. (1981). *Techniques of family therapy.* Cambridge, MA: Harvard University Press.

Minuchin, S., Rosman, B., & Baker, L. (1978). *Psychosomatic families.* Cambridge, MA: Harvard University Press.

Mintz, N., & Schwartz, D. (1964). Urban ecology and psychosis: Community factors in the incidence of schizophrenia and manic-depression among Italians in greater Boston. *International Journal of Social Psychiatry, 10,* 101–118.

Newcomb, S. (1992). Five hundred years of injustice. *Shaman's Drum, 29,* 18–20.

Nichols, M. D., & Schwartz, R. C. (1994). *Family therapy: Concepts and methods* (3rd ed.). New York: Allyn and Bacon.

O'Connor, E. (1971). *Our many selves: A handbook for self discovery.* New York: Harper & Row.

Perls, F. (1969). *Gestalt therapy verbatim.* Moab, UT: Real People Press.

Putnam, F. W. (1989). *Diagnosis and treatment of multiple personality disorder.* New York: Guilford Press.

Rabkin, J. (1979). Ethnic density and psychiatric hospitalization: Hazards of minority status. *American Journal of Psychiatry, 136,* 1562–1566.

Root, M., Fallon, P., & Friedrich, W. (1986). *Bulimia: A systems approach to treatment.* New York: Norton.

Rowan, J. (1990). *Subpersonalities: The people inside us.* London: Routledge.

Satir, V. (1972). *Peoplemaking.* Palo Alto, CA.: Science & Behavior Books.

Satir, V. (1978a). *Your many faces.* Berkeley, CA: Celestial Arts.

Satir, V. (1978b). *The new peoplemaking.* Palo Alto, CA: Science & Behavior Books.

Satir, V., & Baldwin, M. (1983). *Satir step by step.* Palo Alto, CA: Science & Behavior Books.

Schwartz, H. (1986). Bulimia: Psychoanalytic perspectives. *Journal of the American Psychoanalytic Association, 34,* 439–467.

Schwartz, R. C. (1987). Our multiple selves. *Family Therapy Networker, 11,* 25–31, 80–83.

Schwartz, R. C. (1992). Rescuing the exiles. *Family Therapy Networker, 16,* 33–37, 75.

Schwartz, R. C., Barrett, M. J., & Saba, G. (1985). Family therapy for bulimia. In D. Garner & P. Garfinkel (Eds.), *Handbook of psychotherapy for anorexia nervosa and bulimia.* New York: Guilford Press.

Schwartz, R. C., & Perrotta, P. (1985). Let us sell no intervention before its time. *Family Therapy Networker, 9*(4), 18–25.

Selvini Palazzoli, M., Boscolo, L., Cecchin, G., & Prata, G. (1978). *Paradox and counterparadox.* New York: Jason Aronson.

Shakespeare, W. (1974). Much ado about nothing. In G. B. Evans (Ed.), *The Riverside Shakespeare.* Boston: Houghton Mifflin. (Original work performed ca. 1598)

Stone, H., & Winkelman, S. (1985). *Embracing ourselves.* Marina del Rey, CA: Devross.

Stone, H., & Winkelman, S. (1989). *Embracing each other.* San Rafael, CA: New World Library.

Stone, H., & Stone, S. (1993). *Embracing your inner critic.* San Francisco: Harper-Collins.

Suzuki, S. (1970). *Zen mind, beginner's mind.* New York: Weatherhill.

Swift, J., & Letven, R. (1984). Bulimia and the basic fault: A psychoanalytic interpretation of the binge–vomiting syndrome. *Journal of American Academy of Child Psychiatry, 23,* 489–497.

Tomm, K. (1985). Circular interviewing: A multifaceted clinical tool. In D. Campbell & R. Draper (Eds.), *Applicatons of systemic therapy: The Milan approach.* London: Grune & Stratton.

Tomm, K. (1987). Interventive interviewing: Part II. Reflexive questioning as a means to enable self-healing. *Family Process, 26,* 167183.

Tomm, K. (1988). Interventive interviewing: Part III. Intending to ask lineal, circular, strategic or reflexive questions? *Family Process, 27,* 1–15.

Walsh, T. B. (1992). Pharmacological treatment. In K. A. Halmi (Ed.), *Psychobiology and treatment of anorexia nervosa and bulimia nervosa.* Washington, DC: American Psychiatric Press.

Warshaw, R. (1988). *I never called it rape.* New York: Harper & Row.

Watanabe, S. (1986). Cast of characters work: Systematically exploring the naturally organized personality. *Contemporary Family Therapy, 8,* 75–83.

Watkins, J. (1978). *The therapeutic self.* New York: Human Sciences Press.

Watkins, J., & Johnson, R. J. (1982). *We, the divided self.* New York: Irvington.

Watkins, J., & Watkins, H. (1979). Ego states and hidden observers. *Journal of Altered States of Consciousness, 5,* 3–18.

Watkins, M. (1986). *Invisible guests: The development of imaginal dialogues.* Hillsdale, NJ: Analytic Press.

Watzlawick, P., Weakland, J., & Fisch, R. (1974). *Change: Principles of problem formation and problem resolution.* New York: Jason Aronson.

Wechsler, H., & Pugh, T. (1967). Fit of individual and community characteristics and roles of psychiatric hospitialization. *American Journal of Sociology, 73,* 331–338.

White, M. (1989). *Selected papers.* Adelaide, Australia: Dulwich Centre.

White, M. (1991). Deconstruction and therapy. *Dulwich Centre Newsletter, 3,* 21–40.

White, M. (1992). Men's culture, the men's movement, and the constitution of men's lives. *Dulwich Center Newsletter, 4,* 1–21.

White, M., & Epston, D. (1990). *Narrative means to therapeutic ends.* New York: Norton.

Whitman, W. (1959). Song of myself. In J. E. Miller, Jr. (Ed.), *Walt Whitman: Complete poetry and selected prose.* Boston: Houghton Mifflin. (Original work published 1855)

Winnicott, D. W. (1958). *Collected papers.* New York: Basic Books.

Winnicott, D. W. (1965). *The maturational processes and the facilitating environment.* New York: International Universities Press.

Wright, R. (1986, March–April). A better mental model. *The Sciences,* pp. 26–28.

Young, M., & Wilmott, P. (1957). *Family and kinship in East London.* London: Routledge & Kegan Paul.

Zohar, D. (1990). *The quantum self.* New York: Quill/William Morrow.

Index